*About the A*

Dr Robert Erdmann, an American psychologist now living in Tunbridge Wells, has spent the past fifteen years researching the effectiveness of nutritional supplements and using them in his clinical work with patients. He is the technical and managing director of his clinic: Medabolics Limited.

Meirion Jones is a freelance journalist with a particular expertise in health. He is also an accomplished illustrator.

# MINERALS

## THE METABOLIC MIRACLE WORKERS

*The Essential Programme for Maximum Vitality*

Dr Robert Erdmann
and
Meirion Jones

CENTURY

LONDON SYDNEY AUCKLAND JOHANNESBURG

# CONTENTS

First published in 1988 by Century Hutchinson Ltd
Brookmount House, 62–65 Chandos Place,
Covent Garden, London WC2N 4NW

Century Hutchinson Australia (Pty) Ltd
89–91 Albion Street, Surry Hills, New South Wales 2010,
Australia

Century Hutchinson New Zealand Limited
PO Box 40–086, Glenfield, Auckland 10,
New Zealand

Century Hutchinson South Africa (Pty) Ltd
PO Box 337, Bergvlei, 2012 South Africa

Photoset by Deltatype Ltd, Ellesmere Port
Printed and bound in Great Britain by
The Guernsey Press Co. Ltd, Guernsey, Channel Islands

British Library Cataloguing in Publication Data

Erdmann, Robert
Minerals: the metabolic miracle workers:
the essential programme for maximum
vitality.
1. Man. Nutrition. Role of minerals
I. Title II. Jones, Meirion
613.2′8

ISBN 0–7126–1842–2

# Introduction

Our bodies are made up of two fundamentally different groups of substances: organic and inorganic. Organic substances are produced by the chemical reactions of life. They are created, broken down, and recreated in our bodies from the constituents of the food we eat, and the air we breathe forming the dazzling array of molecular structures we need in order to live – nerves, skin, organs and muscles. Organic structures, by their very nature, exist in a state of flux, participating in a continual series of chemical transformations, with one succeeding another like the generations of a family. Organic structures are proteins, vitamins, carbohydrates and fats and thanks to them we can grow and multiply, adapt and evolve.

On the other hand, there is no known way in which our bodies can create or break down inorganic substances. These unchanging chemicals are called minerals. They existed long before organic life first appeared on Earth and will exist long after it has vanished. Yet the role these substances play in sustaining the dynamic, ever changing processes of life is invaluable. Until recently the way that minerals affected our bodies was very poorly understood and as such they tended to be ignored in favour of other nutrients. It is now clear that without them there would be no life at all.

This book explores the vital role that minerals play in ensuring our continued health and wellbeing. It examines their importance in the major structures of the body such as the skeleton, skin, muscles and organs but also shows them at work in the less easily understood but no less important intimate functions of the body; precisely regulating energy levels and water retention, controlling the rate and extent of chemical reactions, and maintaining and coordinating trillions of cell functions every second to ensure that the body works as a single, harmonious organism.

Nutritionists, doctors, researchers and an increasingly health-conscious public are now realizing that minerals are as important to the body as those perennial favourites, vitamins. Even so, our current grasp of the functions performed by minerals in the body is still vague and imperfect and this hazy knowledge often leads us into dietary blind alleys. For example, some nutritionists make arbitrary recommendations about increasing the intake of certain minerals – either through eating more of particular foods or through supplementation – often without fully realizing how these increases might affect the body.

In contrast, this book doesn't recommend the use of particular minerals, as is the vogue, for relieving particular symptoms. What it does is act as a guide to those who want to gain a fuller understanding of the uses and importance of minerals by stressing the way they work as a single, indivisible group. Like proteins and vitamins, fats or carbohydrates, the efficacy of any one mineral in your body depends on existing levels of the others. Each one is affected by the others through complex metabolic interrelationships.

The importance of these relationships is often ignored, but only by understanding them can you hope to unlock effectively the minerals' enormous health enhancing potential. Until now it has been left to a handful of inaccessible text books to highlight this fact while those written with more popular appeal take the easy route by exaggerating the important of one mineral and ignoring the others – as if raising your intake of one mineral could improve your health as simply as raising the treble dial on your record player amplifier could improve the sound.

This book attempts to put the record straight. In it we look at the function and importance of each mineral both individually and, just as importantly, as part of the overall mineral balance. Clearly and concisely we explain how to recognize mineral imbalances, illustrate their causes and list the best ways of correcting them. This holistic approach can achieve marvellous results by showing you how to take advantage of minerals' undoubted therapeutic powers. It is an approach that will help you to achieve strong bones and muscles, good circulation, emotional wellbeing and increased energy levels.

# PART ONE

# MEET THE MINERAL FAMILY

CHAPTER 1

# The Mineral Balancing Act

A woman sits in a small hospital room, slumped in her chair with the docile immobility of old age. She notices a magazine on the coffee table in front of her and bends to pick it up. Leaning forward she extends a trembling hand towards it, so hesitantly that the lasting impression is of someone reaching out to touch a timid animal inch by inch, so as not to scare it away. Instead of picking up the magazine with her fingers she clasps its spine between her palms, lifts it clumsily and drops it onto her lap. Her hands are dry and strikingly white as if she had recently bathed them in chalk dust, the way that gymnasts do before performing. Knuckles the size and shape of marbles have forced her fingers into rigid claws. Arranging the magazine on her lap she prises open the cover and begins to read.

The woman's name is Katherine and, despite her appearance, she is only thirty-two years old. For the past three years she has been suffering from the worsening symptoms of a rare disease called scleroderma. Powerless to halt its advance she has been forced to endure the nightmare of watching and feeling her body literally turn to stone.

Scleroderma is characterized by the growth of calcium deposits in the body's soft connective tissue. Muscles lose their flexibility so that any physical effort quickly becomes exhausting and ease of movement impossible. Tendons seize up causing the joints to grind like sand in the workings of a clock. Worse still is the accompanying pain, the constant dull ache that turns to agony with any sudden movement. Meanwhile the skin itself changes, its soft, pliant quality metamorphosing into something dry and brittle and hard like a thin, encasing layer of plaster.

The immediate response of Katherine's doctor to her illness was to prescribe a diet almost completely free of calcium. The reasoning, after all, was straightforward and seemingly impeccable: if her troubles lay with excessive calcium deposits then her dietary intake of calcium must be too high, in which case a systematic reduction of calcium would probably cure her, or at least halt the progress of the disease. Yet after almost a year on this diet, the only thing that her enforced calcium deprivation has accomplished is to give Katherine the added burden of osteoporosis. Her bones, naturally the largest source and consumer of calcium, have been weakened, the shafts becoming fragile and brittle, easy prey to breakage. Perversely the unwanted calcium deposits continue to grow in her skin and connective tissue, inexorably turning Katherine into a living fossil.

What Katherine's doctor hasn't realized is that her calcium intake is not the cause of her problem. In fact until he imposed her special diet her calcium levels were quite healthy. Paradoxically, the deposits have grown in the soft tissue due to imbalances of other minerals in Katherine's diet.

Many of the most important minerals in our bodies – including magnesium, sodium, potassium and phosphorus as well as calcium – interreact with each other. That is to say, they are intimately connected with each other, both in assisting cell functions and in determining how effectively each is absorbed into the body. Some behave synergistically, helping each other's absorption and functions. Others act antagonistically, hindering absorption and competing for function. In calcium's case function is heavily dependent on a balanced intake of magnesium. Magnesium helps the body to use calcium properly by ensuring that it is distributed to those areas where it is most needed, in the bones and nerve cells, and once there that it is used properly. Without adequate magnesium, calcium would be dumped harmfully in the body's soft tissues. So although Katherine's calcium intake may be well within normal range a magnesium imbalance can quite easily cause her calcium to be metabolized badly. This means that when mineral levels are manipulated to relieve an illness – such as withdrawing calcium in Katherine's case, or even administering additional calcium as is now common practice in osteoporosis treatment – the true source of the problem might be completely ignored.

No one doubts the tremendous effectiveness of minerals in enhancing health. But before they can be used confidently we must understand how these interrelationships work. That's what this book is about. In later chapters we'll be explaining the importance of each mineral to your health, what foods to eat for helping you to relieve particular disorders as well as which supplements you might like to take. But first we'll explain how each mineral works with the next and how they depend upon each other like a set of metabolic cogwheels. We'll be returning to Katherine later in this chapter but before that let's take the first step towards understanding the workings of your body's mineral balance. As far as steps go, it's a long one: fifty billion years into the past.

## An Origin Story

Everything we are, every ounce of protein, fat and bone, not to mention the bricks and mortar our homes are built with, the trees in our parks, the clouds, the wildlife, even the air we breathe, was once, billions of years ago, nothing but clouds of hydrogen atoms floating in space. A hydrogen atom is composed of three parts: a positively charged proton and a neutrally charged neutron which together constitute the nucleus, and a negatively charged electron which orbits the nucleus. The electron is prevented from leaving its orbit by its attraction to the proton in the same way that the two poles of a magnet attract each other.

Over many billions of years these hydrogen clouds coalesced, the gravitational forces they generated massing them into a smaller and smaller volume of space. As happens when any matter is squeezed into a space it is too small for – whether it is a cloud of hydrogen atoms, a kettle of steam or a crowd of football supporters – there was a violent reaction. Such were the forces in the cloud that four adjacent hydrogen atoms fused, resulting in the release of tremendous energy and the creation of helium. Then, through a series of explosions, more electrons began to fuse together and in time each of the elements that make up the world as we know it today were formed. While helium was produced by the fusion of four atoms of hydrogen, carbon was created by six, oxygen eight, calcium twenty, and so on. The explosive energy released by this process is what we call the big bang. When it had finished a hundred or so newly formed elements each produced by the fusion of hydrogen atoms, were scattered across the heavens like seed.

A useful way of categorizing the elements is through the periodic table, a list charting the properties of each element in relation to hydrogen. The lighter an element's atomic weight (that is, the smaller the number of hydrogen atoms that have been fused together to form it) the more abundant it is likely to be. Hydrogen contains a single electron, has an atomic number of one, and is the most abundant element. Most of the major elements which are essential to life fall in the lightest third of the table.

Stepping forward in time to a mere four billion years ago we find ourselves on Earth. The planet is still experiencing the effects of volcanic birth traumas and even now the surface cracks open to emit billions of tons of sulphur and carbon dust into the atmosphere. As the planet cools, steam – a mixture of hydrogen and oxygen – condenses into water and in time the deeper valleys and basins become oceans. Seawater evaporates to form clouds which fall as rain on the land and forms rivers which carry the powdered rock and soil and volcanic dust back to the sea. On the ocean floors violent tremors caused by the cooling, contracting bedrock displace water so suddenly that currents thousands of miles long are forced back upon themselves creating riptides that range across the seabed like hurricanes, ripping up the bedrock and pounding it into microscopic fragments. Tides from around the globe converge and convulse, mixing the debris they carry in an undersea hailstorm. From this, a wide variety of molecules are formed. Sodium particles, for example, will combine with chlorine, magnesium with potassium, calcium with phosphorus. Frequently, each mineral is ground into ever finer fragments between its neighbours. They might settle for a while before being stirred up by a fresh current that tears them into even smaller forms. What we're witnessing is no more or less than the world's first food blender at work, accumulating and preparing the ingredients and conditions for life to start.

Life has two closely related prerequisites: the ability to grow, and the ability to regenerate. There are many different theories both about the exact conditions which obtained when the initial 'spark' of life was generated, and about the source of that spark, and we won't add to them here. Whatever triggered that first leap from inorganic elements to organic, spontaneously growing life forms it happened either in the sea or in the adjoining mud where the conditions were perfect. To exist, grow, and evolve successfully an organism would need as its basic component an element that could bond with itself in long, orderly, repeating chains. Carbon was ideal. Combining with atoms of oxygen, hydrogen, nitrogen and occasionally sulphur, it created strands of amino acids – the building blocks of protein – which in time linked to form the first life forms; tiny viruses and bacteria.

However, in addition to using this small group of elements to assemble protein, these early organisms prospered by using a wide variety of the elements floating in the water around them. Life, in other words, evolved in harmony with its environment, exploiting most of the elements found in the sea or mud. This point is vital, because the most important of these elements in helping life to begin were a collection which we now call minerals.

These minerals were divided into four groups. The first group consisted of all those minerals present in the water in relatively high concentrations and included calcium, magnesium, sodium, potassium and phosphorus. We refer to them today as the gross minerals. The second were the minerals present in much lower concentrations and they included chromium, iron, manganese, molybdenum, cobalt, copper and zinc. Because of their relatively small concentrations the second group are called trace minerals. To give you an idea of the differences in concentration between the two groups the number of calcium molecules contained in each cubic litre of sea water is approximately 800,000 times greater than that of chromium. The third group were those elements in the sea and atmosphere that were necessary for sustaining organic life and which we've already met including hydrogen, nitrogen, carbon, oxygen and sulphur. The fourth group are two elements, iodine and selenium and for convenience sake they are included with the trace elements.

To survive and in time evolve into more complex structures, the first tiny organisms had to utilize every available mineral regardless of concentration (excepting a group of toxins such as lead and mercury that they were unable to use). This growth took place from generation to generation largely thanks to the formation of new and ever more complex organic structures, particularly protein. But the roles that the inorganic minerals played in helping these structures to form was indispensable. Let's see why.

## The Glue of Life

Ultimately every single process of life depends on a series of interacting chemical reactions. For example, to create a molecule of skin protein a single amino acid must bond with many others to form an orderly, repeating protein chain. That bond requires a chemical reaction to 'seal' it. The same is true of a plant absorbing sunlight through its chlorophyll, which enables it to create carbohydrate (its energy source) from carbon dioxide. We call these chemical reactions metabolic pathways. There are hundreds of metabolic pathways in the body serving each of its thousands of requirements (more than 50,000 specialized proteins, for example, are created by metabolic pathways). They are in essence multi-staged chemical reactions which convert the raw materials of life, digested from the food we eat, into custom-built chemicals and structures, like factory assembly lines. At each stage one substance is converted into another. This second substance might itself be used by the body or alternatively be converted into a third. However, this conversion process is anything but a spontaneous, freely occurring reaction as these raw materials are no more likely to convert themselves into a specific substance than a car is likely to assemble itself from its components. Just as the car parts need workers and tools to put them together, so the metabolic pathways need a set of specially designed substances to make them work. These substances are called enzymes.

Enzymes are effectively the molecular cement in the building processes of the metabolic pathways. They bring together the raw materials of the desired reaction, and in doing so help to create a new substance. Unlike cement, though, an enzyme is a catalyst, taking no part in the actual reaction and remaining unchanged by it. Perhaps its role can be compared to that of a party host, who introduces two guests to each other, leaves them to talk and then wanders elsewhere to introduce other guests. In this way a simple enzyme molecule can be used by the body over and over again to 'introduce' many substances to each other. The speed of such reactions is mind boggling. A single enzyme molecule can easily bring about the transformation of half a million reacting cell molecules in less than sixty seconds.

Enzymes, however, don't cause the reactions themselves. Our two party guests might eventually get around to talking to each other without an introduction from their host, and by the same token two substances might actually react together without the interference of the enzyme. Its role is to ensure that the reaction takes place quickly and efficiently, coordinating the reaction rather than causing it. However, this ability shouldn't be underestimated. Because although life, birth and evolution could theoretically have progressed without enzymes it would have been such a sluggish, hit-or-miss affair that it is unlikely even to have reached the amoeba stage by now. Which brings us back to the importance of minerals.

Enzymes themselves are created by metabolic pathways from essential raw materials and in the simplest life forms are composed of amino acids. However, to complete the construction processes of their metabolic pathways they often require the inclusion of other, component chemicals. These chemical extras are known as co-factors and are made up of vitamins and minerals. While most vitamins could be created by the organism itself, rather like proteins, minerals are the odd ones out. They are available to the tiny organisms only from the surrounding environment, the sea in which they drift. Without minerals, in other words, the vitamins and proteins would be unable to function. An example is one of the most important enzymes of all, adenosine triphosphate, which is responsible for releasing energy from carbohydrate. Phosphorus is the most important element in this enzyme and without it cell activity would cease.

The creation of hormones is also highly dependent on the sources of surrounding minerals. While enzymes assist a reaction, giving reacting chemicals the necessary 'push', hormones are chemical messengers which decide the location and rate of chemical reactions. In man, for instance, the thyroid gland secretes the hormone thyroxin to stimulate growth by ordering certain chemical reactions. A major component of thyroxin is the mineral iodine. Adrenalin, the fight or flight hormone, uses three minerals in its manufacture: magnesium, phosphorus and copper. But even in the minute, much less complex organisms of three billion years ago, minerals were vital hormonal components.

## Walling in the Minerals

At this point in our story the tiny animal forms in the sea are little more than wormlike amoebas. Their skins are thoroughly permeable. This means that, simply by moving forward, a constant passage of the mineral-rich water flows through their cells, meeting all their nutritional requirements: providing them with the oxygen, hydrogen, carbon and nitrogen for respiration and growth as well as a balanced, harmonious supply of minerals to aid these organic functions. This process whereby water flows through their cells is called osmosis and is very important to our story. The free flow is guaranteed by the concentration of mineral electrons inside the cell equalling the concentration outside. If, for example, the concentration fluctuates, becoming greater inside than out, then more water must be absorbed in order to dilute the minerals and so rebalance the electrical charge.

By now in our prehistoric ocean there is such an abundance of plant life that the water is becoming clogged like a sargasso sea and, in search of sustenance, the amoebas swim into shallower, fresh-water estuaries around the coasts. Now the mineral content within their cells greatly exceeds that in the mineral-free fresh water. The cells are forced to absorb so much more water to balance the concentration of elements that they literally burst. It is impossible to estimate the numbers of amoebas that die in this way.

In time, though, the animals evolve new mechanisms to protect themselves. First comes an impermeable cell wall to protect them from the danger of osmosis. The importance of this evolutionary step simply cannot be overstated. Up until now the organisms have thrived thanks to their harmonious relationship with their environment. They've been, for all intents and purposes, fragments of living seawater. But by developing their cell wall they have severed the link with their source of life. This leads to new problems as, deprived of their original method of extracting nutrients from the water, they must develop a new way of feeding. So, at the same time as their loss of permeability, they evolve a digestive tract and kidneys both to extract food from the water and to excrete their waste products, and a gill to provide them with oxygen.

During the millions of years in which this is occurring in the sea, plants are colonizing the land. With an atmosphere rich in carbon dioxide they prosper, growing quickly and abundantly by using their magnesium-based chorophyll to convert carbon dioxide to energy. As a by-product massive amounts of oxygen are pumped into the air for the first time. It is now possible for animal life to emerge from the sea.

And so, no longer dependent on the sea for life, the road is paved for the hundred-million-year evolutionary trail from fish to amphibean to reptile to bird to mammal and to man. It's a sobering experience to consider that if the history of life on Earth were measured as twenty-four hours on a clock, beginning with the appearance of the first bacteria at midnight, and concluding with 11.59 p.m. the following night representing the present day, mankind's entire presence would occupy the last fifteen seconds. Our time on Earth seems insignificant yet, in a very real sense, each one of us is carrying our past around with us. Because, even now, our cells depend for their very existence upon a balance and concentration of body minerals which resembles almost exactly the balance and concentration of the seawater as it was at the crucial evolutionary point when the impermeable cell walls first evolved. It is as if the mineral profile has been preserved as successfully as the contents of an Egyptian tomb preserve a way of life that disappeared thousands of years ago. Therefore the mineral demands of our cells today are based on a blueprint three billion years old. In this respect, at least, we are each part of that primordial, turbulent sea.

## Electric minerals

The fact that our bodies contain this concentration of what is, after all, seawater is of enormous importance. For just as the first life forms in the oceans depended on this water for survival, or more specifically on the minerals this water contained, so the fact that we must carry this 'ocean' of minerals around with us today means that it plays a vital role in our lives. The gross minerals – those, you may remember, present in high concentrations – take part in functions concerned with the body's structure, such as growing bone and muscle, as well as determining our energy levels through their involvement with enzymes and hormones. And as ions they help the nerves to carry messages from the brain to every part of the body. But what exactly are ions and how do they work?

Earlier, we introduced electrons as that part of an atom which orbits the nucleus. Put simply, mineral ions are atoms which have lost or gained an electron. A case in point is hydrogen. Since it is the lightest and weakest of all atoms, hydrogen is easily robbed of its electron by heavier, stronger atoms such as oxygen. Because electrons are negatively charged, while the atom overall is electrically balanced, the loss of its electron leaves the hydrogen atom with a positive charge. This positive hydrogen ion is now attractive to any atom in the vicinity that has an additional electron and which is thus negatively charged. The best example of a concentration of hydrogen atoms is in an acid, where the strength of the acid, the pH balance, is determined by the number of positive hydrogen atoms – that is, atoms without electrons – it contains. When you run a wire from an acid to a rich source of electrons such as water, or better still, an alkali, the electrons will surge through the wire into the acid in an attempt to neutralize the positive charge of the hydrogen ions. This passage of electrons creates an electrical current. On a mechanical level this is how a car battery works. But the human body is far more complex than that and by using a variety of different mineral ions – particularly calcium, magnesium, potassium and sodium – each of which are variously trying to attract or repel electrons to balance themselves, it passes millions of different messages up and down the nerve cells in the form of electrical charges.

However, trace minerals, those present in much smaller quantities, are just as important in ensuring cell reproduction, growth, and many other chemical reactions. We'll be looking at the most important of these functions throughout the book, showing how deficiencies or excesses of one or another can quickly disrupt the body's carefully balanced metabolism. We will also look closely at the balances which exist between the minerals themselves. The mineral content of the body, as we've seen, is almost identical to the mineral levels in the sea four billion years ago. Life evolved in this sea by working in harmony with those levels, developing mechanisms to use the available minerals. Sodium chloride was the most abundant mineral available to those early organisms, so many uses for it evolved. Indeed, without sodium today our cells would die. (To illustrate how important a saline environment is, surgeons keep organs in a salt water solution during transplant operations.) Next came the gross minerals like magnesium, calcium and potassium and finally the trace minerals. And these minerals are present in man today in the general ratios as in those primitive organisms.

There is no doubt that minerals can be used effectively to relieve many health problems by restoring the body's homeostatic balance, regulating nerve impulses, providing materials for the metabolic pathways as enzymes and hormones, promoting the health of the cell, and so on. In using minerals, however, many people forget the way that each mineral is related to its siblings. We'll be seeing in Chapter 2 how indiscriminately increasing your intake of a particular mineral can seriously undermine the effectiveness of others, often leading to a chain reaction of hormonal problems that leave the person in a worse state of health than before.

Which brings us back to the unfortunate Katherine. After suffering for three years with no hope of improvement she was finally given an exhaustive mineral analysis. This should, in fact, have been one of the first steps taken by her doctor but as her symptoms pointed to a cut and dried case of calcium excess nobody had thought it worth carrying out. Yet as soon as the results of a hair and intracellular analysis arrived the source of her illness became clear – she suffered from a magnesium deficiency.

Later in the book we'll see in detail how magnesium and calcium affect each other, stimulating the secretion of certain hormones which determine how and where they are used. Without adequate magnesium, for example, calcium will drift around the body like a ship without its crew until it 'runs aground' in soft tissue. This played a major part in what happened to Katherine. However, once the cause of her metabolic problems was clear she was immediately put on a diet high in magnesium with additional supplementation of magnesium together with other important nutrients to promote proper calcium metabolism. Within days ease of movement began to return, allowing her to flex her fingers and move about freely for the first time in three years. Her skin soon cleared up while a measured increase of the calcium in her diet – to strengthen her osteoporotic bones – was conducted in a carefully controlled balance with magnesium. Progress towards a full recovery was slow but, compared with the illness at its worst, her improvement was dramatic.

Sensitivity to the interrelating mineral balances helped Katherine. But what could have caused such a devastating mineral imbalance in the first place?

## CHAPTER 2

# Tipping the Scales

If you were asked to decide what holds centre stage today in the world of nutritional supplementation you would probably suggest vitamins. To support your choice you would only have to point to the veritable mountain of vitamin supplements now available for the increasingly health-conscious public piled up in every colour and flavour of capsule, powder and pill by chemists, health shops and specialist suppliers as they compete for their share of a burgeoning vitamin market.

The variety of mineral supplements, in contrast, is tiny. This is par for the course because in comparison with the body's vitamin needs, which have been exhaustively listed and are well understood, its mineral needs are something most people have only the vaguest knowledge of. Granted, people do know that, for some reason, iron is important for the blood – particularly during menstruation – that zinc has some not quite understood effect on growth, and that calcium may help to protect against osteoporosis. But beyond that? Nothing.

It is only in the last few years that people have begun to realize that mineral deficiencies and imbalances are as widespread, and pose as great a threat to their health, as vitamin depletion. Even so, some experts will argue almost indignantly that mineral deficiencies are impossible, insisting that the human body receives all the minerals it could possibly need from its diet. After all, they say, some minerals such as calcium or magnesium can be found in our food in such high quantities that their levels in the body couldn't possibly become depleted while the metabolic levels of others such as cobalt or chromium are so negligible that we only need to absorb the smallest possible amount from our food to meet all our bodies' requirements. This outlook is dated and misplaced. It is dated for two reasons: firstly, because it takes no account of the damage being inflicted on the soil – our main source of minerals – by modern farming production techniques, and secondly because of the way that modern foods have their minerals stripped from them during processing. And it is misplaced because the simple, indisputable fact of the matter is that thanks to these problems, the mineral levels in our diets are sinking, sometimes at a quite catastrophic rate. Not only does this cause deficiencies of individual minerals but it can undermine the whole mineral balance and lead to chronic ill health.

Happily this decline in our body mineral levels is reversible. By learning how to recognize the symptoms of mineral imbalance, if and when they affect us, we can take steps to eradicate them. We can do this by following a responsible diet of mineral-rich foods and, if necessary, by increasing certain mineral levels by supplementing them with pills or capsules. Examining each mineral in turn, we'll look at the consequences of deficiencies and excesses. We'll see how each one relates to others as part of the overall mineral balance, then put this newly-acquired knowledge to practical use by showing how to fight common mineral-related health problems. But first, in this chapter and the next, we're going to find out exactly how such deficiencies and imbalances can occur; how, for instance, in the face of arguments which say that mineral deficiencies are impossible, Katherine could suffer such prolonged physical and mental torture. These chapters will give you a more complete understanding of the part that minerals play in the world. If you prefer to find out about the individual uses of minerals straight away you can do so by turning straight to Chapter 4 on page 33.

## Coming to Terms

The substances we'll be looking at in this book are divided into two basic categories according to their relative concentrations in the body. One category is called the macro-minerals which, as we saw in Chapter 1, contains those elements which are present in the body in relatively high amounts and are stored mainly in the bones and muscles. They are: calcium, magnesium, phosphorus, sodium and potassium. The second group of minerals are categorized as trace elements, so called because they are present in much smaller, sometimes infinitesimally smaller, amounts. They include iron, zinc, copper, manganese, iodine, chromium, selenium and molybdenum.

Strictly speaking minerals are defined as compounds consisting of an atom of a metal with one or more atoms of non-metal. Examples include sodium (the metal) which combines with chlorine to form sodium chloride, otherwise known as salt. Another example is calcium (the metal) which combines with oxygen and carbon to produce calcium carbonate, or chalk. However, in popular usage the word 'mineral' has developed a much broader meaning. These days it includes not only metallic elements such as calcium and sodium but also non metals such as sulphur and iodine. For simplicity's sake this book has grouped the macro-minerals, trace elements, mineral compounds and non-metals all under the simple collective heading of minerals.

## Mineral Minutiae

Deficiencies of one or more of the minerals may cause illness, physical or mental impairment and even death. This hardly seems credible considering that many of them are present in the body in such small amounts. However, don't forget that since a single enzyme molecule is used many thousands, perhaps millions, of times by the body to affect the same reaction over and over again, the amount of a particular mineral needed to create that enzyme might not be great. Nonetheless, this tiny amount is invaluable for without it the enzyme would not be formed in the first place. Therefore, a deficiency, however small, can be extremely dangerous.

To give you an example, there is approximately 0.002 of a gramme of the micro trace element, chromium, in a body weighing 11 stone. To picture how little this is, imagine holding a single grain of sand in the palm of your hand. You can't feel it. It weighs nothing and is almost swallowed by the creases of the skin. It's less than insignificant. If all the chromium circulating in your body were gathered together into one lump it would amount to no more than this single, solitary grain. Yet this minute amount of chromium plays a vital role in forming a substance that works with insulin to determine how the body uses its blood sugar. It also helps to metabolize fatty acids and cholesterol. Deprive the body of this one, almost invisible, near weightless granule and it will become more vulnerable to diabetes, high blood pressure, atherosclerosis (clogging of the arteries), and heart disease.

## The Mineral Wheel

Although mineral deficiencies cause ill health it is quite wrong to think that simply increasing your intake of one mineral or another will improve it. Too much of a particular mineral can be just as harmful as too little. For example, researchers believe that too much copper causes schizophrenia, while excesses of toxic heavy metals such as mercury and lead can kill. The metabolic imbalances that such excesses cause are due to the antagonistic nature of minerals – in other words, the chemical reactions produced by too much of one partially or completely inhibits the reactions of the other.. Not only does this prevent certain chemical reactions from occurring it also hinders mineral absorption. Each mineral, then, acts on the others in a complex system of checks and balances. If your intake is balanced, and your digestion is working perfectly, all the minerals will be absorbed properly allowing chemical functions to occur normally. But if the ratio of one mineral rises or falls in relation to the others then the overall balance will be disrupted.

For example, an excess of copper antagonizes zinc, iron and phosphorus. Setting zinc and iron aside for a moment, let's see what happens to the depressed phosphorus when its ratio with copper is disrupted. Since phosphorus is one of the minerals used by the body to ensure that calcium is stored properly in the bone, a decline in phosphorus will leave the calcium to circulate wastefully in the blood and soft tissue. This might lead eventually to calcification in the tissue and, without the calcium to replenish its stores, osteoporosis in the bone. If, to combat these symptoms, a doctor recommends raising the victim's calcium intake, then with no means of being absorbed into the bone where it is wanted, this extra calcium will merely exacerbate the problem. And the raised calcium level will also antagonize and depress the intake of magnezium – another important mineral for calcium storage – and zinc, a mineral already antagonized by copper. As you can see, one excess has caused an interlinked chain of mineral imbalances to spread through the body, the first overloaded mineral antagonizing another, and another, and so on. Therefore, whether our intake of one or more minerals is deficient or excessive we are just as likely to fall victim to the symptoms of mineral imbalance. To put it another way, there is an ideal amount of intake for each mineral, determined by the balance between its own importance to the body and the way it interferes with other minerals. This interrelationship is best explained by the diagram on page 19.

As you can see, the minerals maintain a fairly fraught relationship with each other. They get on about as well as the plethora of warring factions in Beirut forced into an uneasy truce by their parity of firepower. The only way to maintain the truce between the minerals is to keep their parity, or ratios, balanced. If one mineral gets the upper hand then the truce breaks down and it starts antagonizing other minerals. In extreme cases this antagonism can lead to imbalances which cause the sort of suffering experienced by Katherine. Even in milder examples imbalances may lead to severe behavioural problems, stress, depression and anxiety, not to mention fatigue and lethargy, or high blood pressure or muscle cramps.

Our bodies are the products of four billion years of evolution. By developing in harmony with the environment evolution has made full use of the available minerals, to finetune our metabolisms. So why are we now experiencing imbalances and fluctuations of intake? The obvious answer is that the mineral levels in the environment itself have changed. How and why are the questions we'll answer next. There are several factors which cause imbalances and we'll look at each in turn.

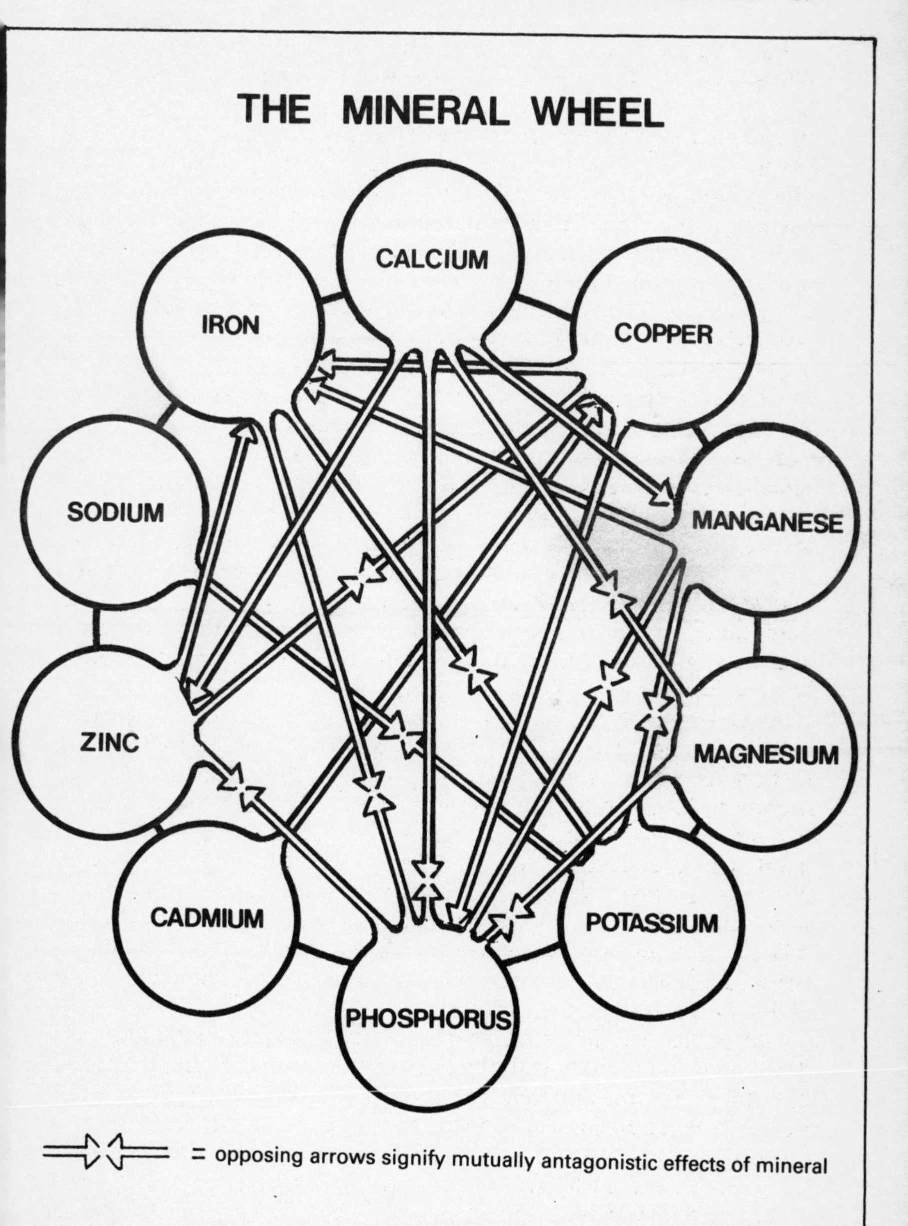
THE MINERAL WHEEL
CALCIUM
IRON
COPPER
SODIUM
MANGANESE
ZINC
MAGNESIUM
CADMIUM
POTASSIUM
PHOSPHORUS
= opposing arrows signify mutually antagonistic effects of mineral

## 1. Stripping the Soil

As we've seen, minerals are inorganic. This means that unlike substances such as protein which can be built from raw materials in our bodies according to specific needs we must obtain our minerals whole from the food we eat. Such food takes the form of certain plants like grains, tubers and fruit, and animal products such as beef, pork and mutton. Ultimately both plants and animals depend for their mineral content on the quality of the soil; the plants feeding on the nutrients in the soil in order to grow, and the animals in turn feeding on plants.

Increasingly, however, the effects of modern farming practices are leading to a decline in soil quality and in particular disrupting the all-important mineral balance. This is because farmers, encouraged by the monetary incentives of agricultural bodies such as the EEC, tend to concentrate on the yield from their fields rather than the quality of produce. Adding concentrations of potassium, phosphorus and nitrogen to the soil as fertilizer causes a field's productiveness to rise abruptly, and at considerable profit to the farmer. Yet, as they behave antagonistically, adding these three minerals inevitably disrupts the ratios between them and the remaining minerals in the soil. The plant's ability to absorb those minerals which haven't been added to the soil decreases as it absorbs more fertilizer, and the overall mineral content of whichever crop the farmer is growing is sent haywire.

By referring to the diagram of the mineral wheel you'll see that increasing phosphorus depresses the levels of absorbed magnesium, calcium, manganese, iron and zinc, while potassium will depress iron, manganese and sodium. The nitrogen, added to the soil as nitrate, depresses sulphur, molybdenum, chromium, iodine and selenium. These deficiencies of minerals in the plants will then be passed on to us when we eat them. In subsequent chapters we'll see how depletions of each mineral affect your health.

Finally, before a farmer's crop – already swollen by the addition of phosphates, nitrates and potassium and polluted by toxic pesticides – is put on the supermarket shelves one last act of mineral stripping will be performed. If it is a plant with a thick, smooth skin such as a courgette, pepper or cucumber it will be sprayed with a chelating agent. A chelator is a chemical which binds to any mineral contained in the organism (chelate means 'to form a claw') and removes it. This gets rid of those minerals near the surface which in nature tend to give the vegetable a slightly greyish hue. The resulting lustrous glow on the plant's skin will lend it an attractive impression of vitality. Nothing could be further from the truth. Robbed of many of its precious minerals the vegetable might have about as much nutritional value left in it as the Emperor's new clothes had gold braid.

So what exactly are the consequences of these imbalances? Let's look at just three of them. Low levels of magnesium – the mineral which suffers most from the farmer's fertilizing techniques – have been linked with a rise in the incidence of cancers, tumours and leukaemia, not to mention contributing to inadequate vitamin C and calcium metabolism, scleroderma (Katherine's problem), heart disease, and muscle and nerve disorders. Iodine depletion, which is caused by excessive nitrates in the soil, can lead to an enlargement of the thyroid gland, also known as goitre. The Earth is ringed with small bands where the soil is iodine-deficient – sometimes as a natural phenomenon, often as a consequence of intensive farming – and in these areas a large, unsightly goitre was much more common than in those areas where iodine was sufficient. Unfortunately these iodine-rich areas are shrinking fast. Finally, a deficiency of selenium – a mineral noted for its anti-oxidant ability –may lead to symptoms that range from dandruff to allergies to skin cancer.

Adding phosphates, nitrates and potassium also has a damaging effect on the soil itself. This is because they kill the soil's inhabitants, tiny microbes which oxygenate the soil and bind it together to give its rich, dark, loamy quality. This destruction reduces the ability of the tiny soil particles to bind together. In time the soil turns to dust and is quickly eroded by rainfall. Many farmers now dig irrigation ditches around their sloping fields to prevent them from simply being washed away by the rain water. Even so, the loss of the mineral-rich topsoil to the rivers and sea is occurring at a frightening pace. One estimate claims that enough topsoil has been lost in Britain since the end of the war (when fertilization began in earnest) to make a plateau fifty metres high with the area of Greater London! And of course, as the topsoil disappears, taking with it the richest soil in terms of minerals, the farmers must apply more fertilizers to the poorer quality undersoil that has been exposed in order to produce the same yield.

## 2. Awkward Plants

Sometimes, even when there is an adequate balance between all the minerals in the soil, prevailing conditions may prevent the plants from absorbing them effectively. For example, decaying vegetation within the soil can produce substances which form compounds with the minerals, rendering them unavailable for absorption by the plant's roots. Some plants also form strong, insoluble compounds from the minerals once they enter the roots. This stops the minerals from being absorbed through the gut when the plants are eaten. Soya beans, for example, often grow in mineral-deficient soils and simply to survive have developed enzymes which inextricably bind what minerals they can get hold of. While this is an effective way of scouring an impoverished soil for minerals it prevents these minerals from being released again once the bean is digested. Phytic acid, a substance contained in rhubarb and cereals also helps these vegetables to hoard their minerals but in doing so hinders mineral absorption into our bodies when we eat them.

## 3. Soil Acidity and Alkalinity

The acidity of the soil also has a major bearing on the availability of minerals for plant absorption. Acidity is measured on a scale called pH that ranges from 0 to 14, on which 0 represents the greatest degree of acidity, or presence of hydrogen ions (those atoms which, as we saw in Chapter 1, have lost their electrons). This decreases logarithmically, reaching neutrality at 7. The numbers 8 to 14 then represent degrees of alkalinity, or declining presence of hydrogen atoms. A strongly acidic soil means that only a limited number of minerals will be made available for absorption. The rest will be hindered by their strong electrical attraction to the acid. These include calcium, magnesium, iron, potassium, manganese, copper and zinc. Likewise, an alkaline soil reduces availability of sulphur and boron. Some minerals, particularly calcium, magnesium and iron, are rendered unavailable by only moderately severe acid or alkaline conditions. This makes the problems of acid rain all the more threatening. Acid rain is created when sulphur, emitted as a waste product from power stations during the burning of fossil fuels, reacts with water in the atmosphere and falls as sulphuric acid. It is a particular menace in Britain, where the authorities, in a mixture of mendacity and cupidity, are reluctant to introduce the stringent laws for reducing emissions that apply elsewhere in the EEC. Acid rain is now so bad that a group of students in North Wales were recently able to run a current through a dense fog on the mountainside, demonstrating that the water droplets were acting like a car battery.

As for alkaline soils they are commonplace wherever the water table approaches the surface of the ground. When a new dam is constructed and the reservoir begins to fill, the water table in the surrounding countryside also rises. This will adversely affect farmers' crops within a vicinity of several miles. Alternatively, if he has sheep grazing on the land the decline in the levels particularly of calcium, magnesium and phosphorus might seriously impair their growth and wellbeing. And if deficiency symptoms remain undetected the depletion will be passed on to humans when they eat the meat. Another cause of a rise in the water table is a decline in Britain's heavy manufacturing industry. Factories were once prodigous consumers of water, and the widespread closures of the 1980s have allowed the water table to rise dramatically, in some cases to within a foot or two of the surface.

### 4. Pollution

Apart from acid rain many other forms of pollution prevent mineral uptake. Particularly dangerous are high levels of lead and cadmium, the waste products of a variety of industrial processes. These two are both highly toxic in their own right, causing hyperactivity, cancer and brain damage. In addition, the deposits that drift down from the atmosphere after being discharged from car exhausts sprinkle the soil with powerful mineral antagonists. Zinc, a mineral essential for promoting growth, resistance to disease, healthy skin and sexual function, is most vulnerable to their interference in plant growth, but these toxins will affect all the minerals to some degree.

### 5. Water

Studies show that people living in hard water areas – that is, water with high levels of magnesium and calcium – stand less chance of developing heart disease, circulatory problems and bone disorders than people living in soft water areas. The hardness of water reflects the state of the soil it has flowed through. Therefore, the harder it is the richer and more nutritious the soil. You can tell the sort of water you have coming into your house by examining the element of your electric kettle for sediment. If there are a lot of grey, plaster-like flakes in the kettle, you have hard water. Many people now use water softeners, which substitute sodium for these other minerals, to reduce this sedimentation. If you are one of them, at the risk of minor inconvenience it would be well worth removing the softener.

These factors are all good reasons for concern about the effects of mineral imbalances. They show how such imbalances are commoner, more widespread, than most of us imagine. However, towering head and shoulders over these examples is an even more prevalent cause of imbalance and deficiency for which each one of us can take individual responsibility and, if we choose, act to put things right. We're talking about the food we eat and it is such a large subject that the next chapter is entirely devoted to it.

CHAPTER 3

# Diets For Deficiencies

In the late sixties scientists knew so little about minerals that the nutritionist Eric Underwood felt confident in writing: 'For the overwhelming bulk of humankind a diet well balanced and adequate in other respects is likely . . . to provide the normal individual with an abundance of all trace elements . . . .' The key words in this passage are 'well balanced'. In the days before food processing gave us refined carbohydrates, canned and frozen vegetables and a dizzying variety of chemical additives the 'well balanced' diet might have been attainable. Nowadays, most diets are anything but balanced. Evidence accumulates daily to show that many of the foods we currently eat and take for granted as staples of our diet are failing to meet even the most basic of our mineral requirements.

Is your diet well balanced? Are you sure that it supplies all your mineral needs? In our highly efficient consumer society you can choose from a monumental variety of foods. Because of this variety there are few shoppers who, standing in a supermarket checkout with a trolley full of meats, fruit and vegetables, bread, sauces, sweets and dairy products, would imagine that their diet was unbalanced. And yet in this sheer dietary profusion, this gluttony of choice, lies one of the greatest causes of mineral deficiency: food processing in the name of convenience. In this chapter we'll see just how unbalanced today's supposedly well balanced diets are.

## Not the Choice We Believe

Some people think that we instinctively choose a well balanced diet. In this respect we're like animals, they say. We pick what we want from the shelves of our supermarkets in the same way that animals pick the foods they know are good for them while rejecting those which they know will harm them. As far as the animal half of the argument is concerned they are quite right. Animals instinctively shy away from poisonous plants or prey. But this only makes the spectacle of humans willingly eating poison every day of their lives all the more absurd.

The fact is that the only time we come close to possessing an instinctive animal-like grasp of what is good for us is when we are babies. Unfortunately, almost as soon as we're born our reactions to the food that our parents offer us are conditioned by many factors that have little to do with instinct or health. By the age of twenty when our eating habits are usually fully formed, the intuition we started with, the intuition that enables us to distinguish between good and bad, has been subverted, blinding us to the fact that much of the food we now happily eat has toxic components.

If you believe that you still retain a clear idea of which foods are good then ask yourself what your basic criteria are for choosing food when you go shopping. Picture yourself pushing a trolley down the aisles of a supermarket. You see a product you want and reach for it from the shelves. Now, freeze your hand in midair and run through all the reasons you might have for picking it. Firstly, how does the way it looks affect your choice? Does the picture of the product on the front of the packet or tin, photographed as a mouth-watering 'serving suggestion', appeal to you? What about the way this picture is incorporated into the overall design of the package, cleverly trimmed, perhaps, into the outline of a casserole dish? Do you like the colours used in the background and the faintly old-fashioned type-face redolent of the age of Mrs Beeton? Whether you are conscious of these factors or not, you would have to be completely insensitive not to respond to at least some of these cultural messages that the packaging transmits to you.

Secondly, once you place it in your trolley you might realize that this product has recently been the subject of an intensive television advertising campaign. Perhaps actors were used to portray a family at the dinner table. They ate the food while engaged in typical family banter that you find not only amusing and sympathetic but strikingly similar to the behaviour of your own family at dinner. By making you identify with their product through its advertising the manufacturers are inviting you to take a personal stake in its success. Choosing it therefore feels that much more natural.

Thirdly, you might have chosen the product because you remember being given it as a child and enjoy fanning the sense of nostalgia. If it is a sweet food you might even remember how strict your parents were about not giving it to you. Admittedly, they did occasionally give in to your pleading and buy it for you, but that only led you into the habit of thinking of it as an extra special treat. Since you thought of the product as something special than it's more than likely that you'll harbour a little of the same feeling now.

Most of our eating patterns, after all, revolve around habit – eating cereal and toast for breakfast rather than lunch, following a main course with a sweet rather than preceding it. And in the same way, if you were brought up on a fairly sweet diet then you are likely to choose foods which include a discernable amount of sugar in their ingredients, or flavour enhancers such as monosodium glutamate if you are used to salty foods. If you were given tinned fruit cocktail as a child the chances are that you'll use it yourself when you make your own meals, rather than chopping up a basketful of fresh fruit.

Which brings us to the fourth factor: convenience. It's been an exhausting day. The balls of your feet are throbbing and you have a persistent ache in the small of your back. Can you really be bothered to spend another hour or so on your feet in the kitchen preparing a meal from fresh ingredients when the contents of three tins, a sachet and two boxes lobbed into the microwave will do the job just as well, and in ten minutes? Probably not. All in all, the old animal instinct hasn't had much of a look-in.

In summary, when you make your choice from the rows of foods available to you, your decision making is almost inescapably influenced by packaging design, advertising, nostalgia, established eating habits, pressure from fussy eating partners, convenience, and taste. None of these have much bearing on knowing instinctively what is good for you. Instead they establish dietary patterns which are anything but 'well balanced'. And in spite of the massive consumer choice we have most of the food which these factors compel us to buy is dangerously unbalanced or deficient in many important nutrients – particularly minerals. But why does so much food suffer from mineral imbalance? There are several reasons and we'll look at each in turn.

## 1. The Empty Calorie Syndrome

Modern processed food contains too much processed sugar and fat. A single ounce of refined sugar has over a hundred calories, an ounce of fat twice that. Yet their calorie content is grossly out of proportion with any other nutritional value that they have to offer. That means our body has to cope with metabolizing these high-calorie-value foods without actually deriving much benefit from them. Unlike natural, unprocessed foods they provide the body with the energy necessary for powering the chemical reactions of life in the form of calories without actually providing any of the raw materials of these reactions. And since figures from the Department of Agriculture and Fisheries show our overall food consumption is declining, while sugar and fat continue to be added to our diets in such high quantities (in Britain we eat an average of 114 lbs of sugar per person per year) they are eaten and absorbed as substitutes for foods which are actually good for us. They are literally empty calories.

The sugar in our food is a particular problem. To achieve the bridal white, free-flowing granular quality of ordinary table sugar, raw sugar is subjected to an extensive and quite extraordinary process of refinement which strips it of almost all of its nutritional value. Because of this, white sugar or sucrose contains less than one tenth the amount of calcium found in raw sugar; one thirtieth of the amount of magnesium and chromium; one fortieth the amount of iron and phosphorus; and one fiftieth the amount of zinc. Other minerals become so depleted by refining that it is almost impossible to measure their presence in white sugar at all. And most brown sugars, such as demerara, are only white sugars with brown colouring.

Even though you might forego spooning refined sugar into your tea and coffee or sprinkling it over your breakfast cereal, you would probably be mistaken in imagining that your sugar intake was low. Most processed foods now contain sugar, using it as both preservative and flavouring. Fruit yoghurts, tins of all kinds – beans, mushrooms, sweetcorn, soups, sauces and fruit – muesli, cereals, jams, breads, cakes, stock, and a variety of packets and frozen foods are all loaded with sugar, as are ales, lagers and wines. You really have to root among the supermarket shelves to find foods that don't contain ounces of these refined, empty calories. Some manufacturers are now belatedly marketing jams made purely from fruit and tinned fruit in their own juices rather than syrup. This appears to be a very halfhearted effort, though, and there are precious few of these products available.

## 2. Flour

Another process which drastically reduces the amount of minerals a food contains is the refining of flour. Until 200 years ago the staple loaf in Britain was made from ordinary, coarse wholemeal flour. However, with the advances in refining techniques which took place during the industrial revolution, the soft, light, white loaves that such techniques produced became a status symbol of the wealthy. It was thought that this more refined bread perfectly suited the more 'refined' classes who were the only ones able to afford it. Inevitably, the desire for white loaves was emulated by the less well off until by the middle of the twentieth century white bread was the only sort of loaf you could buy from many bakeries. This suited the bakers because, since white bread stayed fresher for much longer periods, they could make larger, and thus cheaper, batches of loaves and leave them on their shelves without fear of them going stale. It also suited the consumer as a white loaf not only stayed fresher in the bread bin but could also be cut cleanly without it crumbling. (And if all else failed, the children could make plasticine models from the dough.)

Of course, the question begging to be asked is why white, refined flour makes loaves which stay fresher. The answer is that the chemical reactions that cause a loaf to go stale are, like most reactions, catalyzed by mineral-activated enzymes. Remove the minerals – which is what getting rid of the outer husk from wheat to make white flour does – and you are left with a fluffy white loaf that will stay fresh for ages. Although, since 75 per cent of the minerals have been stripped away this loaf has about the nutritional value of a wad of damp cardboard. To prove the point look at magnesium, of which unrefined flour is one of the most important dietary sources. A frightening 84 per cent is lost in refining. And magnesium isn't the only victim. Manganese loses 88 per cent, chromium and iron 80 per cent, and zinc 75 per cent. The only way to ensure that you get a full complement of these minerals from flour is to eat wholemeal or wholewheat bread. As with sugar, there are many white loaves on the market which have simply been adulterated with caramel to give them a more wholesome, brown appearance. But only wholemeal bread has a full supply of minerals.

The manufacturers of many of the products which use refined grain and sugar go to great pains to replace some of the minerals and vitamins that have been lost. Cereal packets typically carry statements like 'this produce has been enriched with 50 per cent of the average daily intake of zinc, iron and calcium to fortify you for the day ahead'. In fact, if the product really had any nutritional value it would not need 'enriching' in the first place. As it is, these minerals are usually added in forms which are not bio-available, that is, which the body will find next to impossible to absorb, and the only minerals which are likely to 'fortify' you will be obtained from the milk you pour over the cereal.

## 3. Have Mineral, Won't Travel

For supermarkets to sell their goods at such low prices, they must be able to buy from their wholesalers in huge quantities which won't decay during transportation and storage. Most foods, therefore, are stripped of minerals to permit this. Along with flour and sugar, rice is another victim of intensive mineral removal, losing 60 per cent of its mineral content when it is polished. And freezing, another refining process which allows for bulk transport and storage, causes the product to lose their minerals when they thaw. Vegetables, for example, are blanched immediately before being frozen, losing about 25 per cent of their minerals in the process. As they are defrosted the minerals are simply drained off in the water. When meat is thawed much of the iron it contains seeps away and the same thing happens to frozen fish which loses its precious iodine.

## 4. Lost in cooking

Even when you are preparing unprocessed, wholly fresh food, it is easy to cause an unnecesary loss of minerals. Minerals cannot be destroyed but they can be unwittingly discarded. Many vegetables contain a large proportion of their minerals near the surface – either in their skins or in their outer leaves. We saw briefly in the last chapter how chelating processes can remove minerals from these outer areas to make them appear brighter than they really are. The same sort of depletion can be caused simply be tearing off and discarding the outer leaves or peeling the skin and throwing it away. In addition, soaking vegetables such as potatoes in water and then boiling them causes them to discharge their minerals into the water. Even worse is when the water – now virtually a mineral soup – is simply poured into the sink. Instead it should always be kept for use as a stock or to make a soup, helping you to get the full benefit of the minerals in your food.

With so many factors adversely influencing your diet it is easy to see how we can reach a state of mineral deficiency: the cumulative effects of mineral imbalances in the soil which are passed on to fresh vegetables and meat are only exaggerated by the nutritional shortcomings of processed food. Bearing this in mind you would think that the British health authorities would do their utmost to let us know about the deficiencies in our food. The least they could do is to set out a comprehensive guide, listing the recommended daily allowance (ROA) of each mineral in our diets. Yet, astonishingly, Britain has

*Recommended daily allowance*

| | | UK | | US | |
|---|---|---|---|---|---|
| | | Adults | Pregnant women | Adults | Pregnant women |
| Potassium | mg | none | none | 3750 | 3750 |
| Sodium | mg | none | none | 2200 | 2200 |
| Chloride | mg | none | none | 3400 | 3400 |
| Calcium | mg | 500 | 1200 | 800 | 1200 |
| Phosphorus | mg | none | none | 800 | 1200 |
| Magnesium | mg | none | none | 350 | 450 |
| Iron | mg | 12 | 15 | 10 | 48 |
| Zinc | mg | none | none | 15 | 20 |
| Copper | mg | none | none | 2.5 | 2.5 |
| Iodine | mcg* | 140 | 140 | 150 | 150 |
| Selenium | mcg | none | none | 125 | 125 |
| Chromium | mcg | none | none | 125 | 125 |

* microgramme

one of the lowest nutritional standards of any western country. DHSS guidelines exist for only three minerals: calcium, iron, and iodine. See how our standards compare with those of the United States. As you can see, it is very much up to the individual in Britain to decide upon their own mineral requirements and look out for possible deficiencies for themselves. The spirit of free enterprise indeed.

The watchword when trying to evaluate our mineral needs for ourselves is 'sensitivity': sensitivity to our reasons for buying the food we eat to guard against being seduced into making purchases for spurious reasons such as nostalgia and flashy packaging; sensitivity to a food's mineral content so that what we do buy is nutritious; and sensitivity to the way we prepare our food so that our diets really can become 'well balanced'. Making yourself aware of how easily mineral imbalances occur and the precautions you must take to avoid them, is the first step towards ensuring full health for you and your family.

Still, you might be unlucky enough to take all the precautions in the world and still fall victim to deficiencies. How you can test for them is the basis of our next chapter.

# PART TWO

# GROSS MINERALS: THE MISAPPLIED MIRACLE WORKERS

CHAPTER 4

# Beware: the Calcium Myth

Of all the minerals none is currently receiving so much public attention as calcium. For many it has become the dietary equivalent of a western gunslinger. Just as any gunslinger worth his salt will singlehandedly beat the outlaw gang that has terrorized his town, so calcium will vanquish a host of harmful illnesses, helping the victim to rediscover their health and wellbeing. Many dieticians, nutritionists and health writers cover acres of print extolling the properties of this one mineral, elevating it with their extravagant praise to the status of a nutritional wonder substance. In America, books on calcium are so numerous that they almost constitute their own sub-genre, while the handful that have so far appeared in Britain are surely only the first trickle of an eventual deluge. Whatever your problem, they say, whether you suffer from insomnia, depression, excessive irritability, muscle cramps, high blood pressure, heart disease or osteoporosis, then simply by raising your calcium intake you can prevent or even reverse these conditions. At least, that is the claim. It is not one with which the PR people of the delighted dairy and calcium-supplement industries feel inclined to disagree.

At first glance the arguments which the calcium supporters advance to back their claims are impressive. But they fail to realize, or choose to ignore, important facts which show that simply raising your calcium intake, either through your diet or specific supplementation, while ignoring its complex interaction with other minerals, can have little or no health-enhancing effect. Worse, it may itself lead to other health dangers. Considering the sweeping claims of the calcium lobby and the role that calcium is assuming in today's health-conscious – or alternative-health-conscious – society it is important that we pause and put its true benefit into perspective. We should examine the whole picture rather than getting carried away by the avalanche of pro-calcium propaganda. So let's look at the full calcium story.

## Calcium's Role in the Body

To begin with, everyone agrees that calcium is one of the body's most important substances. It is also one of the most abundant, making up about 2 per cent of overall weight – or, on average, about 3 lbs. In various forms it is indispensable for a host of bodily functions. It is one of the three minerals for which the department of health in Britain has decided to give a recommended daily amount (RDA), specifically 500 mg, and 1200 mg for pregnant or lactating women.

## Bones and the Calcium Tide

Your bones and teeth contain 99 per cent of all the calcium in your body. It combines with phosphorus to form a compound called calcium phosphate and together the two minerals are incorporated into the bone where they bond with a latticework of fibrous protein. This protein acts rather like the chicken-wire armatures that sculptors employ to support their clay models. The bonding process between mineral and protein is essential, for bone provides the anchorage and levers for muscles; without bone we simply wouldn't be able to move. It protects organs and supports the entire body.

When we think of bone we tend to picture it as an unchanging, rocklike substance. Many people are therefore surprised when they discover that the whole skeleton is in a constant state of flux, so dynamic that the changes within it almost seem tidal. The calcium phosphate that gives the bone its hardness is continually forming, dissolving and being reformed. New calcium phosphate deposits are usually built into the protein matrix along the bone shaft while older material is flushed away in the blood to be used for other purposes or excreted by the kidneys in the urine. This constant bone refurbishment allows for growth in the young and ensures that adult bones remain strong and resilient. In this way, an average of 700 mg of calcium moves into and out of the bones every day.

Interestingly, to work properly, the process needs the assistance of gravity. This allows for the necessary forces and stresses of leverage to be brought into play which in turn stimulate bone mineralization. Hospital patients who have to spend long periods in bed are often found to suffer from bone calcium loss. Similarly, during the American skylab mission of the seventies, despite vigorous exercise, the absence of gravity made the astronauts' bones lose on average 200 mg of calcium a week. Back on Earth, researchers have found that half an hour's exercise a day using the levers of the bones and muscles is invaluable in helping to keep calcium in the bones.

The constant calcium renewal performs several different roles. Firstly it keeps the bones healthy, removing any imperfections that might form as well as ensuring that any breakages will be repaired. Secondly, it allows the body to use the skeleton as a calcium bank.

When any of the calcium that circulates in the blood isn't required elsewhere, rather than excrete the calcium, the body deposits it into the bones which store it like a current account in a bank. Then, when a need for calcium outside the bone does arise, it is withdrawn. (The hormonal mechanisms used by the body for moving calcium into and out of the bones, both for storage purposes and to help keep the bones healthy, are crucially important to our story. We'll be exploring them in depth later in the chapter.) Away from phosphorus and the bones, calcium becomes soluble. This allows it to circulate freely, and be quickly and easily transported. So what sort of needs is calcium likely to meet outside the bone?

## Calcium and Nerves

One of its most important duties is in helping to control nerve and muscle excitability. To do this it is used in ionic form by the nervous system to regulate the transmission of a special set of nerve impulses. We saw in Chapter 1 how different mineral ions – atoms with an unbalanced positive or negative charge – are used by the body to transmit messages in the form of electricity along the nerves. Different minerals transmit different messages. A nerve cell's reaction to a given stimulus, such as heat, cold or pain, consists of a two-part response; irritability (the initial response to that stimulus) and conductivity (the passage of this response through the nervous system to the brain or vice versa). Calcium's job includes keeping these two reactions in check, ensuring that the strength of nerve irritability and conductivity never exceed the strength of the original stimulus – in other words, it prevents the nerves from overreacting.

A number of factors may prevent sufficient calcium from reaching your nerve cells. Excess dietary fibre is one, as it binds with calcium in the small intestine and prevents it from being absorbed as well as it might. Phytic acid – a substance found in grains – as well as too much fat in your diet have the same effect. Alcohol, too, prevents your body from utilizing calcium by causing the kidney to excrete it in the urine.

When there is an inadequate number of calcium ions in the nerve cells, they quickly become oversusceptible to stimuli. In time this would cause the person to become tense, irritable, bad-tempered and highly sensitive to those distractions that most of us take in our strides: the noise of a car, perhaps, or banging a knee on a table leg. Even the sheer tactile quality of everyday objects such as cutlery or newspapers can become unbearable. The classic example of this form of oversusceptibility is the unpleasantness of pre-menstrual tension. When a woman's ovaries are least active, immediately before her period, the change in her hormonal balance causes the level of ionic calcium circulating in her blood to drop. This starves the nerves of the calcium they need to regulate their responses and plays a major part in causing a woman's nervousness, short temper, insomnia, depression and nausea. Studies show that a large proportion of the women arrested for violent crimes are found to be in this calcium-deficient state.

## Calcium and the Muscles

Soluble calcium also assists normal muscle contraction, keeping the body well toned and in readiness for immediate activity. Inadequate muscle calcium can be a factor in the loss of muscle control, resulting in facial twitches, or an inability to coordinate movements and pick up objects, as well as a loss of tone, aching muscles and joints, and an increasingly flaccid body. This loss of muscular control may also lead to heart problems as contractions become irregular, causing the heart either to 'miss a beat', or alternatively beat much more rapidly than it should.

Calcium also helps the blood to clot. It achieves this by liberating a clotting agent, thromboplastin, from the blood platelets – clotting cells. Thromboplastin is a crucial component of the metabolic pathway that creates the clotting protein, fibrin, and without it almost any wound would cause the body to bleed to death. In addition, calcium plays a major role in forming and activating a number of enzymes that assist muscle functions, protein formation and digestion.

From what we've seen so far, calcium is obviously an important and versatile nutrient. This versatility is due to a unique partnership that it enjoys with a protein called calmodulin. This protein, which is found in every organism from protozoa to man, is, in effect, a metabolic adaptor plug. It has four separate connecting sites which can each be used by a maximum of four calcium ions. This results in the possibility of sixteen different calcium/calmodulin combinations. Very simply that means that calcium can be linked into many more different metabolic pathways, thanks to this protein, than any other mineral. Consequently, it has important roles in cell division, enzyme secretion, smooth muscle contraction, nerve regulation and blood coagulation. It is also used as an intracellular messenger, helps to manufacture amino acids and releases hormones. Bearing this versatility in mind is it any wonder that calcium has attracted so much attention?

But, despite this, there are countless vitamins, minerals and proteins that our bodies need in order to live. What makes calcium special? What has caused the unrivalled interest in this one mineral, currently eclipsing all other nutritional aids in terms of popularity? There is a one word answer to this question: osteoporosis.

## The Magnificent Obsession

Put simply, osteoporosis is a disease which is characterized by a decrease in bone mass. Affecting the jaw bone, spine, and pelvis particularly severely, it causes the bone to soften and become porous, leading to brittleness and eventual fracture. These breakages inevitably take a longer time to heal. Significantly, osteoporosis occurs when more calcium is withdrawn from the fibrous protein matrix of the bone than is deposited. In effect, the calcium tide goes a little further out each time than it comes in again. Osteoporosis is usually impossible to detect – even by x-ray – until at least 30 per cent of all the calcium has been withdrawn from the skeleton. And, technically, it is only said to be present when a person suffers a fracture. Such a fracture might, incidentally, be caused by something as simple as stepping off a kerb. Osteoporosis is generally recognized as an age-related disease. One in three women over the age of fifty five and men over sixty have suffered a fracture as a direct result of this disease.

We'll be examining the problems of osteoporosis in Chapter 15. For the moment, let's look at the contents of the Pandora's box that concern with osteoporosis has let loose: namely, today's widespread obsession with calcium as a nutritional supplement.

Deciding that osteoporosis was ostensibly a loss of calcium from the bone, nutritionists began to speculate on the possible benefits of raising a patient's calcium intake, both by increasing the quantities of calcium-rich foods in their diet and by administering calcium supplements. After all, they thought, if the major symptom of the problem is calcium deficiency, then raising the calcium levels will surely help to relieve it. This is the very straightforward reasoning that provided the fuel for calcium's commercial success; the spark that ignites the flame was provided in the late seventies by a recommendation from the United States National Institute of Health which stated that the daily calcium intake should be at least 1000 mg and as high as 1500 mg for pregnant, lactating or post-menopausal women. This compared with the actual recommended daily allowance in the US of 800 mg and in the UK of 500.

Health writers, catering to an increasingly nutritionally aware and health-conscious public – a public unwilling simply to accept conventional medical assertions about osteoporosis being an unavoidable part of old age – quickly jumped aboard the calcium bandwagon. One columnist, writing for a prominent health magazine, declared sweepingly: 'If you want to ensure optimum health, just be sure to get enough calcium.' 'It's the world's best kept youth secret,' said another. It was claimed to be a cure not only for osteoporosis but for hypertension, irritability, insomnia and heart disease. Calcium was heralded as a conveniently ingested, naturally acting cure to these problems, and calcium mania quickly gathered a momentum of its own. Health supplement companies rushed to market their own calcium tablets, food manufacturers 'fortified' products such as flour and orange juice with calcium (and even created an instant calcium whip) and dairy groups used the fact that milk, cheese and yoghurt have high calcium contents as the basis for their high-profile advertising campaigns. In 1983 a third of all nutritional supplements sold in the States were calcium based. America went calcium crazy, and Britain is now in the early stages of the same thing. Just look for proof at the newly-marketed high calcium milks such as 'Calcia' and 'Vital'. In fact the Advertising Standards Authority recently rejected a claim by Unigate, the producers of Calcia, which claimed that their calcium-enriched milk helps to prevent osteoporosis.

However, the simple logic on which all this is based – namely, if your bones start losing calcium simply increase your intake – is now being shown as unsound. Certain facts about human metabolism are starting to emerge which expose the calcium fad for the self-inflating myth it is. This whole question of calcium deficiency is in fact related to a complicated series of interactions, a metabolic clockwork mechanism in which various hormones, vitamins and minerals depend upon each other to maintain the body's calcium levels and bears little relation to the actual level of calcium intake. Most health writers have the very best of motives but they have singularly ignored the importance of these interactions, focusing instead on misguided, and possibly dangerous, blind alleys.

Let's look at the true story, as we see it, of the way your body effectively utilizes calcium. Vitamin D, firstly, is crucial in ensuring that calcium is absorbed from the small intestine into the body. This is because it activates the production of a special 'binding' protein whose job it is to chelate, or latch onto, calcium molecules and literally carry them across the gut lining. Without this protein, calcium molecules would be unable to pass. Vitamin D deficiency has been related to poor bone and teeth formation, bone softening and retention of phosphorus in the kidneys. Researchers believe that these symptoms of deficiency are caused largely by the fact that when there is inadequate vitamin D in the body calcium absorption decreases.

Vitamin D, also known as calciferol, is the substance that our bodies create from the ultraviolet light in sunshine. Many people living in hot, sunny climates, and whose diets have been found to contain much less calcium than British diets, nevertheless have a perfectly adequate calcium content in their bones, blood and cells. This is because, as they are exposed to more sunlight, their vitamin D levels are that much higher, hence they can absorb the calcium which is contained in their diets much more efficiently. This is one example which shows that calcium levels in the bones do not have to depend on the amount of calcium contained in the diet. To be fair, most health commentators and supplement manufacturers tend to mention this point when praising calcium, recommending that their readers always take calcium in harness with vitamin D.

However, even when calcium has successfully passed into the body the mineral still depends upon a complex interaction of hormones to help store it in the bones. Without this interaction you could ingest all the calcium and vitamin D you wanted yet bone absorption wouldn't improve at all. The calcium would simply stay in the blood while the bone itself might even start to dump calcium. And worse, if the calcium isn't deposited in the bones, but rather builds up in the blood and soft tissue, serious health problems may ensue. For it is enormously important that the level of serum calcium – the calcium in the blood – remains within narrow limits. Too little serum calcium results in problems such as the nervous disorders we've looked at; other, equally serious problems can occur when there is too much. The results of excessive serum calcium might include calcification of soft tissue, particularly arteries and veins where the calcium will begin to collect on the blood vessel walls leading in time to arteriosclerosis and high blood pressure; tendons and muscles might also begin to calcify leading to stiffness, cramping and joint pains; in extreme cases calcification will occur in the skin, too, leading to loss of pliability, cell death and premature ageing; and the body's energy levels will drop dramatically. This, in effect, was what happened to Katherine, the woman whose case we looked at in Chapter 1. Originally her calcium intake had been normal, yet calcification still occurred in the soft tissue. Then, when calcium was reduced in an attempt to combat the scleroderma, it merely weakened her bones.

Don't forget, all these problems can be caused by excess calcium circulating in the blood, calcium which many people take in the first place to strengthen weakening bone. So what do we have to do to ensure that the calcium is sent to where it is needed – to the bones – and that the calcium levels remain within their narrow acceptable boundaries?

For the answer we must examine the method the body uses to deposit and withdraw calcium from the bones. This continual process – the ebb and flow of the calcium 'tide' – depends to a large extent on two hormones: calcitonin (CT) and parathyroid hormone (PTH). If we think of the bones as the current account of a bank, then calcitonin is the body's paying-in book. It makes sure that calcium is deposited in the bones and in doing so prevents the excessive uptake of calcium by the vulnerable soft tissue. PTH, on the other hand, functions rather like a cheque book. When a need for calcium arises outside the bones PTH secretions withdraw the required calcium from the bones, thereby encouraging the uptake of calcium by the soft tissue. In this way all the body's functions such as regulation of nerve transmission and blood clotting are maintained. Therefore it is the way these two hormones work together that maintains the body's bone and serum calcium balance. What are the factors that keep this balance, ensuring, for example, that PTH secretion doesn't exceed CT?

Quite simply the body depends, in turn, upon other substances to regulate these hormonal secretions. The female hormone, oestrogen, for one, plays a major role in keeping PTH production down. In other words, oestrogen, as well as determining a woman's fertility, is also responsible for helping to keep calcium in the bones. So when oestrogen production declines during the menopause, the secretion of PTH is slowly allowed to rise leading in time to a progressive release of calcium from the bones into the cells. This is why oestrogen replacement therapy is often used to treat osteoporotic women (more of which in Chapter 15).

But other substances are involved in maintaining the calcitonin/PTH balance as well. The most important of these is the mineral magnesium. Few people give a thought to magnesium. Yet healthy body levels of magnesium, like oestrogen, stimulate calcitonin production and at the same time suppress the production of PTH. Low magnesium, on the other hand, allows the levels of PTH to rise. Increasing one's magnesium intake will actually help the body to make better use of its existing calcium resources.

However, this now brings us full circle back to the issue of calcium supplementation. Unfortunately, calcium and magnesium are antagonists. This means that as far as ingestion into the body is concerned, they must compete tooth and nail with each other for absorption. The more of one mineral you absorb the less you'll absorb of the other. Increasing your calcium intake, as is the vogue, inevitably depresses magnesium. With less magnesium available, PTH secretion rises and calcium is withdrawn from the bone. So what is magnesium and how does it affect calcium and the body? That's what we're going to look at in the next chapter.

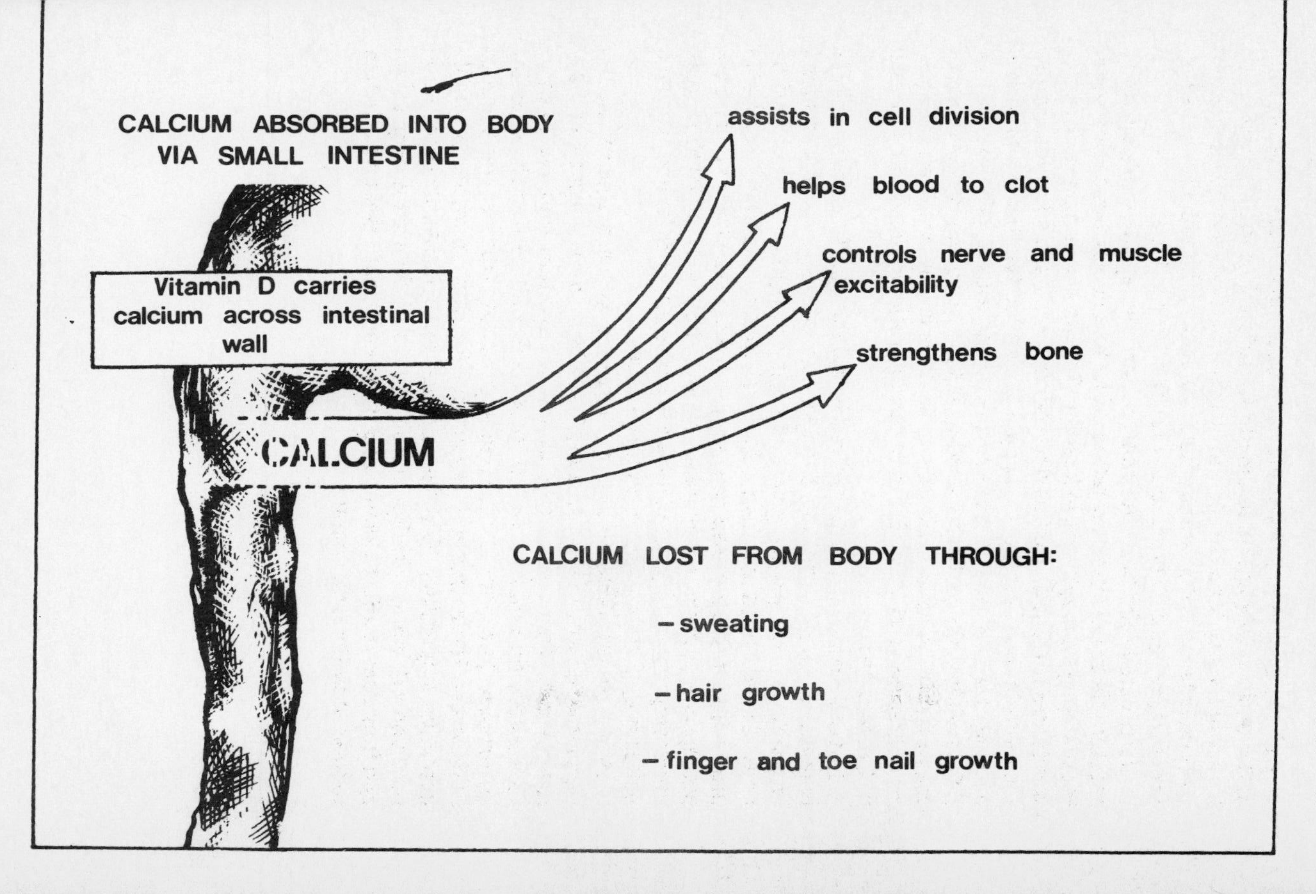
CALCIUM ABSORBED INTO BODY
VIA SMALL INTESTINE
Vitamin D carries
calcium across intestinal
wall
CALCIUM
assists in cell division
helps blood to clot
controls nerve and muscle
excitability
strengthens bone
CALCIUM LOST FROM BODY THROUGH:
– sweating
– hair growth
– finger and toe nail growth

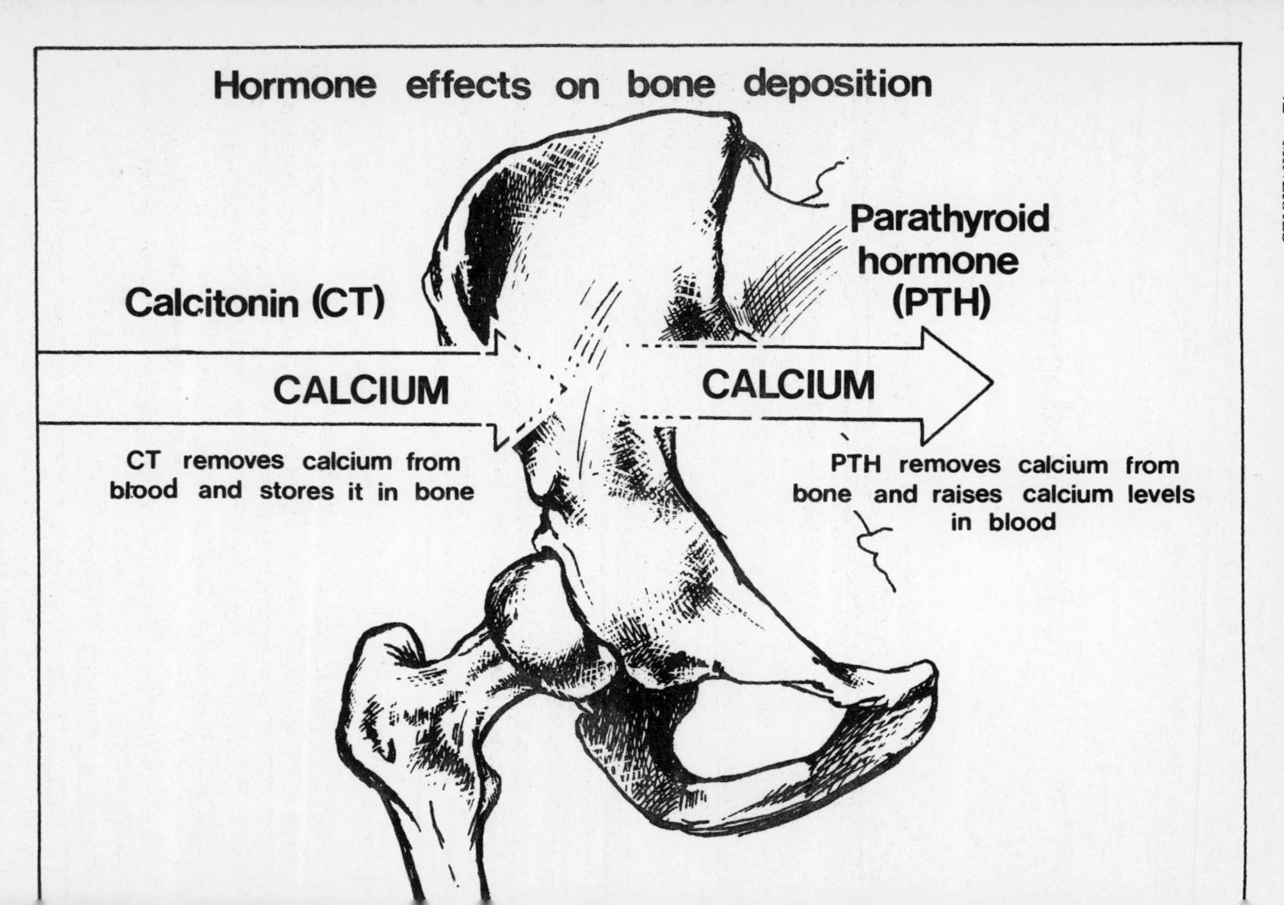
Hormone effects on bone deposition
Calcitonin (CT)
CALCIUM
CT removes calcium from blood and stores it in bone
Parathyroid hormone (PTH)
CALCIUM
PTH removes calcium from bone and raises calcium levels in blood

CHAPTER 5

# Meritorious Magnesium

It is worrying that the British health establishment recommend a daily calcium intake of 500 mg (and articles, books and dairy producers imply that the more of it we consume the healthier we'll become) without setting a matching requirement for its dietary twin, magnesium. Consult any British table of nutrients and in the amount column next to magnesium you'll see the word 'none'. It is as if the powers-that-be regard magnesium as a non-substance, not seeing fit to acknowledge that it serves any useful purpose in the body. Are they suggesting that you can happily follow a magnesium-free diet and expect to live a full and vital life? If so they are making a scandalous assumption. And were anyone to take them at their word it would prove fatal. Magnesium is one of the most important of all nutrients (organic or inorganic). It is of course the dietary prerequisite for ensuring that calcium is distributed properly in the body and in this chapter we'll see exactly how it does this. However, its functions extend far beyond that one job. In this chapter we'll see just how far.

## Magnesium and the Body

An average adult body contains about 30 grammes of magnesium, 70 per cent of which is stored in the skeleton. Unlike the ever-fluctuating calcium, the magnesium in our bones exists in a more permanent, unchanging state. Our main interest, therefore, lies with the remaining 30 per cent or so not in the bone. Most of this is kept inside the cells of the body's soft tissue – again in marked contrast to that fraction of calcium that is not stored in the bone which circulates in the blood and lymph fluid.

Under normal conditions, approximately 50 per cent of the magnesium you eat is successfully absorbed by the small intestine, although this figure will vary greatly with the conditions. Alcoholism as well as high sugar intake, protein and fat consumption and the use of diuretics will reduce the amount absorbed. Health disorders such as poor digestion and low stomach acidity, epilepsy, kidney trouble, hyperthyroidism and high blood pressure also depress the amount of magnesium successfully absorbed. High levels of dietary phosphorus in particular actively prevent its absorption. Since phosphorus is highly concentrated in red meat, cheese and eggs, while the best magnesium sources, on the other hand, are found in less popular foods such as nuts, grains and beans, the magnesium balance often falls victim to an excessive dietary intake of phosphorus.

Because of so many obstructions the average daily magnesium intake for many adults drops from its optimal level of between 300 and 400 mg to as little as 150 mg. Tests suggest that as many as 70 per cent of the population are magnesium-deficient. Unlike minerals such as calcium and iron, however, magnesium deficiency is hard to trace unless a doctor or nutritionist specifically looks for it. Sadly, very few are likely to waste their time searching for a deficiency in a mineral which, without a recommended daily requirement, can never be officially recognized as such.

## A Tale of Two Minerals

As we've seen, the parts played by magnesium and calcium in sustaining the body's metabolism are inseparably linked. So the wildly differing perceptions of their usefulness – calcium as the efficacious cure-all, magnesium as an unimportant and anonymous constituent of our food – is utterly misguided. However, despite the fact that they need each other, calcium and magnesium will always compete for absorption. And as the mechanism the body uses to absorb magnesium is easily upset, when the calcium intake rises, magnesium is bound to drop, unless you increase your magnesium intake too. And, as we'll see, the two minerals are so closely interlinked that many of the symptoms of magnesium deficiency are mirrored in those of calcium. Let's see how.

## Magnesium in the Nerves

To start with, a magnesium deficiency upsets nerve and muscle functions. The results of this will range from nervous tics such as a mildly embarrassing eyelid that won't stop twitching to large-scale, uncontrollable muscle tremors, overexcitability, stress and convulsions. You may remember we described many of these same symptoms in Chapter 4 as consequences of calcium deficiency. The reason why these problems resemble each other so closely is that both minerals work to maintain efficient nerve cell function – magnesium ions inside the cell, calcium ions outside.

When they are balanced these ions regulate the electrical activity of nerve impulses as they are relayed from the brain to whichever part of the body is to receive the message. Calcium, as we know, is the stimulator – regulating the degree of 'irritability' – magnesium the relaxor. In this respect they work in the same way as those metal transformers you see outside large buildings. A transformer's job is to receive electricity from the national grid and reduce its voltage, literally transform it, to manageable proportions before relaying it into the building. If for some reason the transformer breaks down and is unable to reduce the grid's electrical potential, the wiring in the building will be overloaded and fuse. In the same way, if the calcium/magnesium cell balance is disrupted by insufficient magnesium then the strength of the messages passing into the cells will be too great and the cells themselves will become overloaded with an unprecedented charge of 'stimulation' from the calcium outside the cells.

The results of this overstimulation will include the loss of muscular control that we've already mentioned, for while calcium causes muscular contraction, the muscles can only relax again if they have sufficient magnesium. It will also lead to an oversusceptibility to the sensory messages that our nerves carry to the brain, causing over-reactions to everyday sensations: we might experience the dizziness and nausea of vertigo simply by standing at the top of a flight of stairs; we might find the sound of a doorbell shocking and annoying; even the thought of having to phone the garage to complain about a bill might lead to unreasonable anxiety. All this will be due to our nervous systems 'fusing' thanks to insufficient magnesium. And as the magnesium/calcium imbalance worsens so a victim's nervous instability will increase. Depression, anxiety, severe mental disorders, such as schizophrenia, and suicide have all been attributed to loss of magnesium.

## Magnesium and the Blood

Chronic magnesium deficiency has also been found to result in heart and circulatory disorders. This too is caused by an imbalance between the two minerals in the nerves. By reducing the effect of a nerve message to the muscles, and thus causing them to relax, magnesium works like the brake pedal of a car to calcium's accelerator. Magnesium precisely determines the strength of the muscle relaxation in the same way that careful pressure on the brake pedal will reduce your speed in a flow of traffic. Suffering from a magnesium deficiency in the muscle cells is like experiencing a brake failure as you approach a traffic jam. Put simply, the muscles will dangerously overrespond.

Low magnesium allows calcium to contract the muscles without any opposing relaxation.

Many of the most important muscle cells control the circulatory system and an immediate result of this failure to relax is vasospasm, a violent contraction of the blood vessels. This causes high blood pressure and interrupts the blood supply. Severe cramping in the chest (angina) and limbs is caused when tissues are starved of the oxygen which should be distributed to them by the blood. Tests conducted at the University of Wales in Cardiff show that heart disease victims contain 30 per cent less magnesium than the average. To back this up, a group of men suffering from chronic hypertension experienced an 11 per cent decrease in their blood pressure when they were given magnesium therapy. In addition they reported lower pulse rates and more regular heartbeat.

Magnesium is also used by the body to give strength and rigidity to the lining of blood vessel walls. A loss of magnesium here will result in weakness that is certain to be aggravated by the consequence rise in blood pressure and the violent muscular spasms that ripple along the walls, and tiny ruptures are a common result. In turn these ruptures make ideal spots for the blood cholesterol to settle and build up. Eventually this may lead to arteriosclerosis, fibrillation and blood clotting. Blood clots in the vessels are one of the major causes of heart attacks and strokes. Conventionally they are blamed on high cholesterol levels but, insists the biochemist Richard Passwater, there is simply too much emphasis today on blood cholesterol when the incidence of heart disease could be cut in half simply by supplying the potential victims with adequate magnesium.

## The Magnesium Balance and Bone

Of course, calcium and magnesium also influence each other heavily when it comes to determining the structure of bone. We saw in Chapter 4 how calcium is stored in the bone but can be withdrawn when necessary thanks to the counterbalancing action of two hormones, calcitonin – which is primarily concerned with depositing calcium in the bones – and parathyroid hormone (PTH) – which is used to withdraw the calcium. The relative levels of these hormones depend not only on the amount of calcium in the body but also on magnesium.

Calcitonin, the bone-storer, is secreted when the serum levels of either calcium or magnesium are high. However, a careful analysis of research indicates that calcitonin release probably depends more on a good amount of magnesium than on calcium. Therefore, although your body's serum levels of calcium may be quite high, creating a need for calcitonin release so that it will be stored safely in the bones, this calcium will continue to circulate in the soft tissue as long as your magnesium levels are depressed. In this case only the addition of a magnesium supplement, or increasing your dietary intake of magnesium, will ensure that enough calcitonin is produced to store the calcium in your bones.

Alternatively, since calcitonin and PTH oppose each other, and since both low magnesium and low calcium will stimulate PTH, in the final analysis it may be the ebbing magnesium levels which prove more effective at causing PTH secretion. Therefore, even if your calcium levels are normal in your bones and serum, a magnesium deficiency will cause the body to start dumping calcium from the bones into the soft tissue where it may cause extreme harm. Repeated tests have shown that an adequate calcium, low magnesium diet leads to calcification in the soft tissue, heart and muscles, and skin mottling, as well as bladder and kidney stones, both caused by calcium buildup.

A test conducted over five years at the University of Boston proves the effectiveness of magnesium. In this test, a large group of people prone to recurrent kidney stone trouble caused by excesses of calcium in the soft tissue were made to follow magnesium-enhanced diets. By the end of the five-year observation period kidney stones had decreased by an incredible twelvefold. And if further proof is needed we won't get a more graphic demonstration of the interrelationship between calcium and magnesium than those truly awful problems of Katherine's that we saw in Chapter 1, primarily resulting from an inadequate magnesium intake. The fact that calcium needs magnesium like a fish needs water is a point that needs repeating until everyone takes notice.

## Magnesium on its Own

So far we've seen magnesium purely in terms of its relationship with calcium. Magnesium, however, also performs a variety of vital functions in the body independent of its metabolic double-act. Perhaps its most important solo role is that of a co-factor in the creation of an estimated 80 per cent of all the body's enzymes. Enzymes, you may remember, are the catalysts of every chemical reaction in the body, bringing the various raw materials obtained from your diet together in order to custom build specific proteins, release energy from starches and dispose of waste products.

In particular, magnesium is a vital enzyme co-factor in the cells for the manufacture of specific proteins from deoxyribonucleic acid – DNA. This substance is, in effect, a molecular blueprint for the entire body contained whole in each one of the body's 100,000 billion cells. Each new act of growth and regeneration must refer to these master plans. They ensure that whatever the body needs, whether it is a molecule of eyeball tissue or leg muscle, the newly created structure perfectly conforms to a pre-existing model. The process of replication is carried out with the help of strands of ribonucleic acid (RNA) or ribosomes, molecular copies of the particular section of DNA that is being referred to. The raw materials to be used in assembling the finished product are matched with the pattern on the ribosome, following each of its genetic instructions, and then bonded together by enzymes. The process finishes with a spanking new molecule ready to be incorporated into the body.

Each step of this process, creating a ribosome from the parent DNA, assembling the raw materials on the ribosome, then bonding them together, depends upon magnesium-derived enzymes. Any enzyme deficiency could seriously hinder the faithfulness of the reproduction, and nutritionists now speculate that a magnesium deficiency could result in cell mutations and even cancer. Indeed, a recent experiment in America using rats showed that magnesium deficiency can cause leukaemia. And Dr P. Bois at the University of Montreal has shown that magnesium deficiency increases the incidence of spontaneous cancer growth. Bearing this in mind it is reasonable to expect that even a relatively mild magnesium deficiency could lead to tissue that heals poorly, greater susceptibility to degenerative diseases and premature ageing. Many nutritionists, in fact, now suggest that magnesium would make an effective anti-wrinkling supplement.

## Causes of Magnesium Deficiency

Magnesium depletion can be caused by many factors. Stress is one of the most common. When we respond to stress the adrenal gland secretes adrenalin, a hormone which has an excitory effect on the body, preparing it for action. The heartbeat quickens and blood is directed away from the gut, where it helps with digestion, to supply the heavy muscles with the oxygen that helps them to cope with increased physical demands. At the same time brain activity and awareness is heightened. Adrenalin is constructed from a metabolic pathway that uses magnesium as a co-factor. The more stress a person finds himself under, the more adrenalin he will need in order to cope with it. This will in turn consume more magnesium. Since stress is now so common in modern, everyday life, many people are finding themselves victims of nutritional deficiencies. A long list of nutrients is involved in the metabolic pathway that creates adrenalin, including several amino acids, but magnesium is as important as any of them. The irritability you feel when you are under stress, your tendency to overreact in the most innocuous of circumstances, and the high blood pressure that you might experience as a result, are all common symptoms of stress and are thought to be closely related to magnesium depletion because of magnesium's ability to regulate and tranquillize the nerves. This is why magnesium is used as a natural tranquillizer, helping to reduce tension and relieve insomnia.

Alcoholism also leads to an acute loss of magnesium, causing wasteful spillage into the urine. Alcohol-related magnesium deficiency plays a major part in rupturing a heavy drinker's blood capillaries, both through a rise in blood pressure and a loss of strength and pliability in the vessel walls. At one end of the scale this causes the almost comical, Falstaffian redness of an alcoholic's nose and cheeks as the blood from the burst vessels suffuses through the skin; at the other it can lead to loss of sensation, cramping and, in extreme cases, make amputation necessary.

Laxatives and diuretics will also cause magnesium depletion. This is particularly important for pre-menstrual women, who may be suffering from the characteristic symptoms of cramping, irritability and short-temper and are caused by magnesium and calcium deficiency. Since water retention is one of the most unpleasant symptoms women often use diuretics to relieve the uncomfortable bloated sensation. The fact that by doing so they will also unwittingly excrete important amounts of magnesium and calcium, and thereby aggravate their symptoms, is a fact that few doctors have recognized. If a diuretic is taken during the premenstrual phase, magnesium and calcium supplements should always be taken with it to safeguard against any loss.

## How Much To Take

Dr Emanuel Cheraskin, a doctor with an enormous amount of experience in this field, suggests that the ideal magnesium content of a healthy illness-free adult is somewhere between 300 and 500 mg. A separate recommendation is that adults should take 6 mg daily for every kg of body weight. For a person weighing 70 kg (11 stones) this works out at 420 mg and fits in well with Dr Cheraskin's theory. In America the RDA is 350 mg a day, rising to 450 mg for pregnant women, while in Russia it's 500 mg, rising to 925 mg. The average diet in Britain contains about 120 mg per 1000 calories and since few diets rise much over 2000 calories the amount of magnesium we get from our food is obviously not sufficient to meet our needs. This is especially true if we eat a lot of processed food as modern techniques strip away the magnesium as if it were unwanted wallpaper. Traditionally, nutritionists recommended a calcium-magnesium intake in the region of a 2:1 ratio. However, since magnesium is now looked upon as a problem nutrient some researchers suggest raising one's magnesium intake to match calcium 1:1. If you choose you can do this by referring to the food tables on page 58 and altering your diet accordingly, or through supplementation (see pages 172–4).

But there's one final member of our cast which has been waiting patiently in the wings for its cue. And with the next chapter it makes its long-awaited entrance.

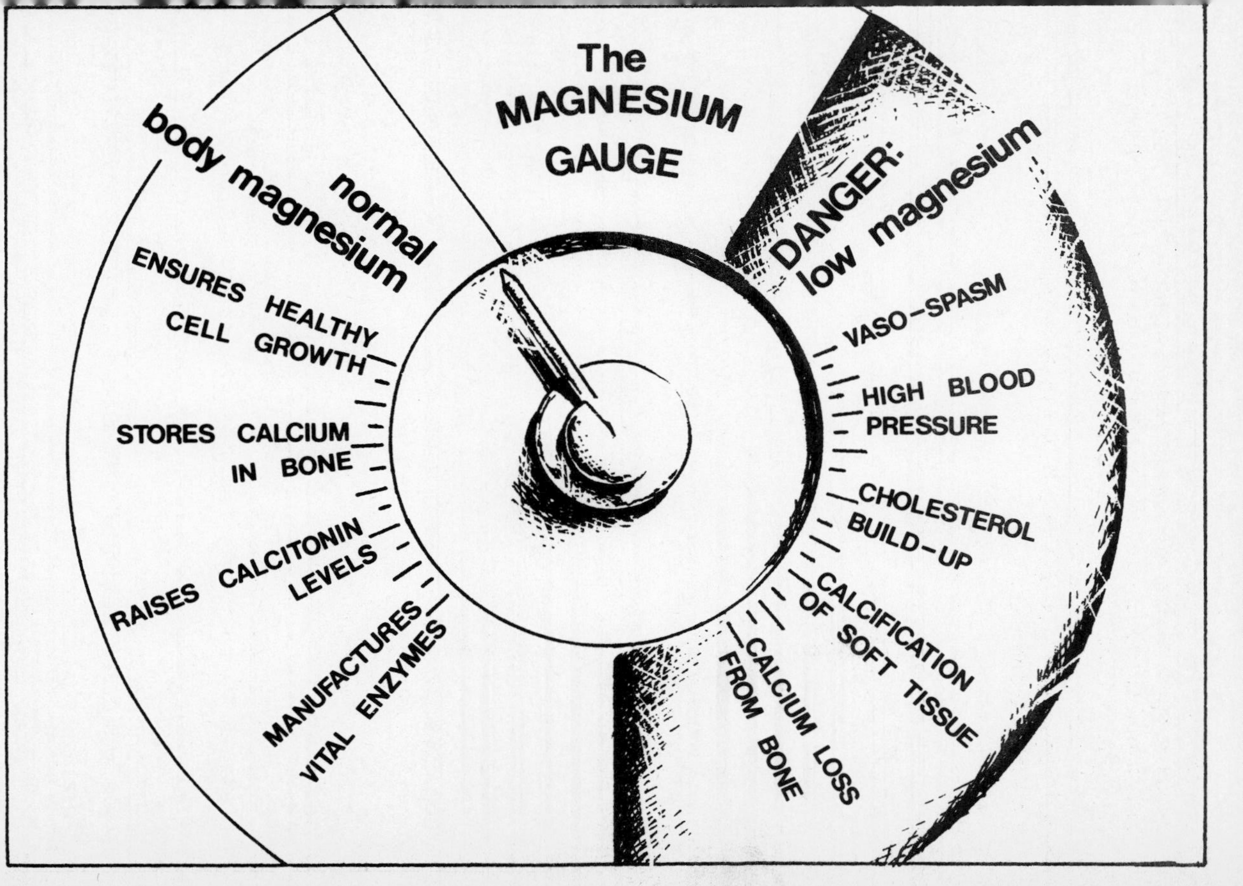
The
MAGNESIUM
GAUGE
normal
body magnesium
ENSURES HEALTHY
CELL GROWTH
STORES CALCIUM
IN BONE
RAISES CALCITONIN
LEVELS
MANUFACTURES
VITAL ENZYMES
DANGER:
low magnesium
VASO-SPASM
HIGH BLOOD
PRESSURE
CHOLESTEROL
BUILD-UP
CALCIFICATION
OF SOFT TISSUE
CALCIUM LOSS
FROM BONE

CHAPTER 6

# Inseparable Phosphorus

We've gone to some length in the last two chapters to stress the way that calcium and magnesium affect each other. We've done this because the vitally important metabolic relationship of this pair is commonly ignored – an oversight that can cause a lot of unnecessary suffering. Unfortunately, now that we've established the importance of a good calcium/magnesium balance it is time to throw everything into a fresh state of confusion by introducing a third important mineral, phosphorus. Like magnesium, phosphorus plays a crucial role in determining how well calcium is absorbed and distributed in the body. Unlike the metabolically unassuming magnesium, though, phosphorus is a biochemical bully, which, if allowed, will antagonise its mineral partners and trigger a number of chronic disorders.

Phosphorus is second only to calcium in terms of its abundance in the body; the average adult containing between 600 and 900 grammes or about 1 per cent of overall body weight. In common with most minerals there is no British RDA but in America the recommended daily intake is 800 mg, rising to 1200 mg for pregnant and lactating women.

## The Attractions of Phosphate

Eighty per cent of all the phosphorus in the body is contained in the bones and whenever we speak of calcium's role in bone manufacture we should always include phosphorus in the same breath. This is because the two are stored together in the bone as a compound called calcium phosphate. Phosphate is the name for the compound formed when an atom of phosphorus combines with four atoms of oxygen, resulting in the creation of a strong, negatively charged molecule. This means, since many chemicals in the body, including calcium, are positively charged, that they are very strongly attracted to the negatively charged phosphate. Because of this, phosphate – and thus phosphorus – participates in more metabolic pathways than any other mineral in the body.

It is the highly 'attractive' phosphate which, by linking with calcium, lends it the ability to bind itself to the protein matrix of the bone. Thanks to this, adequate phosphorus is as important in contributing to the hardness of teeth and calcification of bone as, in their own ways, either calcium or magnesium. For example, even though your magnesium intake might be excellent – encouraging calcitonin secretion to store calcium in the bones – without adequate phosphorus the calcium simply wouldn't have any means to attach itself to the bones.

Since phosphorus is so abundant in our food, a deficiency of this order is very unlikely. (In fact, as we'll see later, we are in far greater danger of falling victim to an excess of phosphorus.) The only possible cause of phosphorus deficiency is thought to be a loss of stomach acid resulting from a regular programme of antacid supplements. This, incidentally, also affects calcium and magnesium. Phosphorus, like most minerals, is best digested and absorbed in the acid environment of the stomach and upper end of the small intestine. Consequently, antacids may cause a phosphorus depletion and this can be recognized by symptoms of weakness, lethargy, fatigue, loss of appetite and depression.

You might also lose the digestive hydrochloric acid from your stomach as a natural part of the ageing process. Ironically, it is the elderly, the group most in need of raising their phosphorus intake to match the decline in their powers of absorption, who, because of the high calorie content, tend to eat less of those foods which contain phosphorus in abundance such as meats and eggs.

If the phosphorus depletion is severe it will lead to calcium excesses in the blood. For without adequate amounts of phosphorus to form the compound calcium phosphate, the calcium would be prevented from mineralizing in the bone. Circulating redundantly in the soft tissue, this wasted calcium would in time trigger the symptoms we are now familiar with of calcification and imbalance such as osteoporosis, loss of muscle control and strength, trembling, convulsion, high blood pressure, arteriosclerosis and heart disease.

## Phosphorus Excesses

Most of the recognized phosphorus-related illnesses are not caused by deficiencies but stem in fact from having too much phosphorus in the body. Considering how abundant it is in our diets, this is a problem that can occur easily. Let's see what sort of mischief it causes.

The combination of phosphate with calcium is one of the most useful reactions, making calcium available for incorporation into the bones. There is so much phosphate in the body that it combines with other minerals as well and unfortunately the results aren't always so happy.

For example, when the same reaction occurs with magnesium it produces a compound that renders magnesium completely unable to perform its functions as an enzyme co-factor and regulator of nerve impulses. Not content with that, phosphorus also antagonizes magnesium, competing with it for absorption across the wall of the digestive tract.

Another damaging consequence of absorbing too much phosphorus is a state called secondary hyperthyroidism. Quite simply this is an illness in which the parathyroid gland – a crucial component of the body's calcium absorption mechanism – secretes more parathyroid hormone (PTH) than the body needs. PTH, you may remember, is one of the two hormones (the other being calcitonin) which determines the balance between calcium absorption into and withdrawal from the bones. PTH is secreted when there is a shortage of calcium in the body's soft tissue as its job is to withdraw calcium from the bone.

However, by stimulating PTH secretion when there is no call for it, excess phosphorus can cause serious illness. One such illness is reaching almost epidemic proportions in the United States. There the phosphorus intake is estimated to be the highest in the world. Red meat (an American staple) has a phosphorus to calcium ratio of 20 to 1; junk food is loaded with phosphorus additives; and soft carbonated drinks, of which the average American drinks more than forty gallons each year, are pumped full of phosphates to decrease their acidity. Because of such high levels of dietary phosphorus, Americans of all ages are finding themselves unwitting victims of chronic calcium loss. In the elderly this takes the form of osteoporosis, high blood pressure and other common symptoms of calcium imbalance such as skin calcification and mottling. In the young it leads to a loss of calcium from the most heavily calcified bone in their bodies – the jaw – and a consequent rise in the incidence of tooth diseases. Their gums become painfully inflamed while their teeth loosen in their sockets and slowly rotate free of their jaws. Ironically the carbonated diet drink products which, thanks to their sugar-free formulas, have been hailed by their manufacturers as a significant step towards weight control and the prevention of tooth decay, are nothing of the kind since the phosphorus they contain is as big a culprit as the sugar. In Britain soft drink consumption per person is barely a third of that in America. Even so Britain is considered a prime target by the slavering soft drinks companies as they search for promising markets to expand into. So watch out.

From these examples we can see that phosphorus is both a blessing and a curse. It can stimulate the unnecessary secretion of PTH, haul calcium needlessly from the bone, and obstruct magnesium. Then again it is an essential factor in clamping calcium firmly in the bone.

## Phosphorus and Energy

Like all substances natural to the body's metabolism phosphorus performs many important roles and one of these is so fundamental to existence that without it life would never have begun. We already know that phosphate is one of the most useful molecules in the body thanks to its remarkable bonding ability. The same quality which sees calcium fixed firmly into the bones is employed in creating the body's most indispensable biochemical molecule, a substance called adenosine triphosphate or ATP for short. This molecule is responsible for supplying the body with all the energy it needs.

We obtain energy from the fats, proteins and carbohydrates (starches) that we eat. These foods are digested in the gut and absorbed into the body as sugars, transported to the cells and broken down into minute structures called mitochondria to produce carbon dioxide and water. The energy released by this process is measured in units called calories and is the power source of life, providing the body with the fuel it needs to reproduce, repair, grow, think, see and move. Since the dietary supplies of energy fluctuate – after all, we eat sporadically and even then our meals are often unbalanced – and since the energy released from splitting the sugars is too great to be used all at once, the body relies on ATP to conserve the energy like a battery. In this way ATP prevents too much energy from surging through the cells at one time by storing what isn't immediately needed, while also being able to release this stored energy for use by the body when the dietary sources are lower. Without this phosphate-derived, energy-regulating molecule the body simply couldn't live.

## But How Much?

Having established the importance of phosphate in our bodies, how much phosphorus is healthy? Like every mineral it is not only the overall amount of phosphorus that is important but also how much we eat of it in relation to the other elements. On the one hand a good phosphorus level will help to clamp calcium into the bones in addition to forming ATP and performing a variety of other functions in the body. On the other, excessive amounts will cause calcium to spill out of the bone as well as preventing the body from absorbing magnesium. Therefore, our intake needs to be in a ratio to the other minerals which enables it to meet all the body's requirements without there being enough left over to cause serious imbalances.

Discovering the optimal ratio is a problem that has occupied scientists and dieticians for years. Many respected experts have come to strikingly different conclusions. Tests conducted on animals in laboratory conditions point to a ratio roughly equivalent of two parts phosphorus to one part calcium as ideal for promoting bone mineralization. Western diets, on the other hand, show ratios as wide of the mark as 6:1 and with fifty times more phosphorus than calcium contained in meat it is easy to see how this ratio is arrived at. Some nutritionists have suggested using calcium supplementation together with a high calcium diet to increase the ratio to as high as 2:1 in calcium's favour, backing their ideas up with blood tests to show a high level of calcium retention in people on these diets. Measuring mineral levels from blood tests, though, is a notoriously inaccurate guide to calcium retention and simply noting a high calcium level in the blood is not a guarantee of good bone absorption. No matter what ratio you choose, remember that you also have to consider the calcium-magnesium relationship too. To this end, the tables and charts on the following pages should be of some use to you.

## At-a-glance guide to Calcium, Magnesium and Phosphorus

### *A. Calcium Metabolism*

| Calcium: | Inadequate calcium metabolism: |
|---|---|
| Assists in bone formation | Causes osteoporosis; calcification of soft tissue (including skin, muscles, and organs) |
| Regulates nerve excitability | Causes oversusceptibility to stimuli; anger; depression; violence |
| Helps muscle contraction in limbs and circulatory system | Leads to loss of muscle control; irregular heartbeat; loss of muscle tone; flaccidity |
| Assists blood clotting | Lengthens bleeding time |
| Activates a variety of enzymes for muscle function, protein formation, digestion and cellular messengers | |

### *B. Magnesium Metabolism*

| Magnesium: | Magnesium deficiency: |
|---|---|
| Assists with muscle and nerve relaxation and helps prevent over-stimulation. Counter-balances excitory effect of calcium | Causes loss of muscular control leading to tremors; inability to relax; oversusceptibility to stimuli; vertigo; depression; anxiety; mental disorders; high blood pressure; vasospasms; angina |
| Strengthens blood vessels | Creates a greater chance of blood-vessel wall rupture; calcification; arteriosclerosis; fibrillation; heart attack; stroke |
| Stimulates bone-storer, CT, and depresses bone withdrawer, PTH | Increases PTH secretion and therefore more calcium to be withdrawn from bone; leads to calcification of soft tissue (such as kidney stones, arteriosclerosis and scleroderma) and osteoporosis |
| Works as enzyme co-factor in manufacture of structural protein, enzymes and hormones | May result in cell mutations and cancer, greater susceptibility to disease and stress, and premature ageing |

### *C. Phosphorus Metabolism*

| Phosphorus: | Phosphorus excess: |
|---|---|
| Links with calcium, helping it to join to the bone; maintains hardness of bones and teeth | Increases secretion of PTH (bone withdrawer) leading to chronic bone loss, calcification of soft tissue and tooth diseases<br>Competes with magnesium for absorption and renders it unavailable to the body |
| Participates in the creation of ATP, a molecule which stores energy ready for release if and when it is needed | |

*Calcium content of food in milligrammes per 100 grammes*

| | |
|---|---|
| Kelp 1093 | Oranges 41 |
| Goats' milk 129 | Celery 39 |
| Buttermilk 121 | Cashews 38 |
| Yoghurt 120 | Barley 34 |
| Sunflower seeds 120 | Brown rice 32 |
| Milk 118 | Cauliflower 28 |
| Olives 106 | Onion 27 |
| Broccoli 103 | Fresh green peas 26 |
| Cottage cheese 94 | Cooked lentils 25 |
| Spinach 93 | Asparagus 22 |
| Romaine lettuce 68 | Pineapple 17 |
| Dates 59 | Chicken 12 |
| Prunes 51 | Beef 10 |
| Artichokes 51 | Bananas 10 |
| Cabbage 49 | Apples 7 |

*Magnesium content of food in milligrams per 100 grammes*

| | |
|---|---|
| Kelp 760 | Raisins 35 |
| Wheat bran 440 | Fresh peas 35 |
| Almonds 270 | Potato with skin 34 |
| Molasses 238 | Crab 34 |
| Brazil nuts 225 | Bananas 33 |
| Peanuts 175 | Broccoli 24 |
| Tofu 111 | Cauliflower 24 |
| Spinach 88 | Carrots 23 |
| Brown rice 88 | Celery 22 |
| Shrimps 51 | Chicken 19 |
| Sweetcorn 48 | Green pepper 18 |
| Cheddar cheese 45 | Tomatoes 14 |
| Avocados 44 | Milk 13 |
| Parsley 41 | Pineapple 13 |
| Cooked beans 37 | Mushrooms 13 |

*Phosphorus content of food in milligrammes per 100 grammes*

| | |
|---|---|
| Brewers' yeast 1753 | Beef liver 352 |
| Wheat bran 1276 | Brown rice 221 |
| Brazil nuts 693 | Eggs 205 |
| Almonds 504 | Chicken 239 |
| Cheddar cheese 478 | Beef or lamb 150 |

Cooked lentils 119
Mushrooms 116
Fresh peas 116
Milk 93
Yoghurt 87
Brussels sprouts 80
Prunes 79
Parsley 63
Asparagus 62
Cauliflower 56
Potato 53
Spinach 51
Avocados 42
Carrots 36
Tomatoes 27
Bananas 26
Lettuce 26
Onions 26
Olives 17
Apples 10

*Comparison of mineral content in a selection of foods in milligrammes per 100 grammes*

| | Magnesium | Calcium | Phosphorus |
|---|---|---|---|
| Almonds | 270 | 234 | 504 |
| Apples | 8 | 7 | 10 |
| Avocados | 45 | 10 | 42 |
| Bananas | 33 | 8 | 26 |
| Beef | 21 | 10 | 150 |
| Broccoli | 24 | 103 | 78 |
| Cabbage | 13 | 49 | 35 |
| Carrots | 23 | 37 | 36 |
| Cauliflower | 24 | 25 | 56 |
| Cheese | 45 | 750 | 478 |
| Chicken | 19 | 12 | 239 |
| Dates | 58 | 59 | 63 |
| Grapes | 13 | 16 | 20 |
| Kelp | 760 | 1093 | 240 |
| Milk | 13 | 118 | 93 |
| Onions | 12 | 27 | 36 |
| Oranges | 11 | 41 | 20 |
| Pineapple | 13 | 17 | 8 |
| Raisins | 35 | 62 | 101 |
| Spinach | 88 | 93 | 51 |
| Sweetcorn | 48 | 3 | 111 |
| Tomatoes | 14 | 13 | 27 |
| Wheat bran | 490 | 119 | 1276 |

*Relationship between minerals and hormones during bone absorption*

Calcitonin (CT):
1. Decreases blood calcium
2. Blocks uptake of calcium by soft tissue
3. Deposits calcium in bone
4. Deposits phosphorus in bone
5. High calcium levels stimulate CT production
6. High magnesium levels stimulate CT production
7. Low magnesium decreases CT production
8. Oestrogen stimulates CT production

Parathyroid hormone (PTH):
1. Releases calcium from bones
2. Releases phosphorus from bones
3. Increases blood levels of both minerals
4. Encourages uptake of calcium by soft tissue
5. Low tissue calcium stimulates PTH release
6. Low magnesium stimulates PTH release
7. Oestrogen decreases PTH production

Calcium:
1. High vitamin D increases calcium absorption
2. Low vitamin D decreases calcium absorption
3. Calcium competes with magnesium for absorption
4. High serum calcium decreases absorption of magnesium
5. Low serum calcium increases absorption of magnesium
6. Calcium metabolism is partially regulated by magnesium, partially by calmodulin
7. The body can adjust well to low calcium intake

Magnesium:
1. High magnesium suppresses PTH production
2. High magnesium stimulates CT production
3. Low magnesium stimulates PTH production
4. Low magnesium suppresses CT production
5. It is difficult for the body to adjust to low magnesium intake

Phosphorus:
1. Combines with magnesium and other minerals rendering them unavailable
2. Phosphorus is synergistic with calcium absorption
3. PTH increases phosphorus release from bones
4. CT increases phosphorus deposition in bone
5. Excessive phosphorus leads to calcium loss from the bone

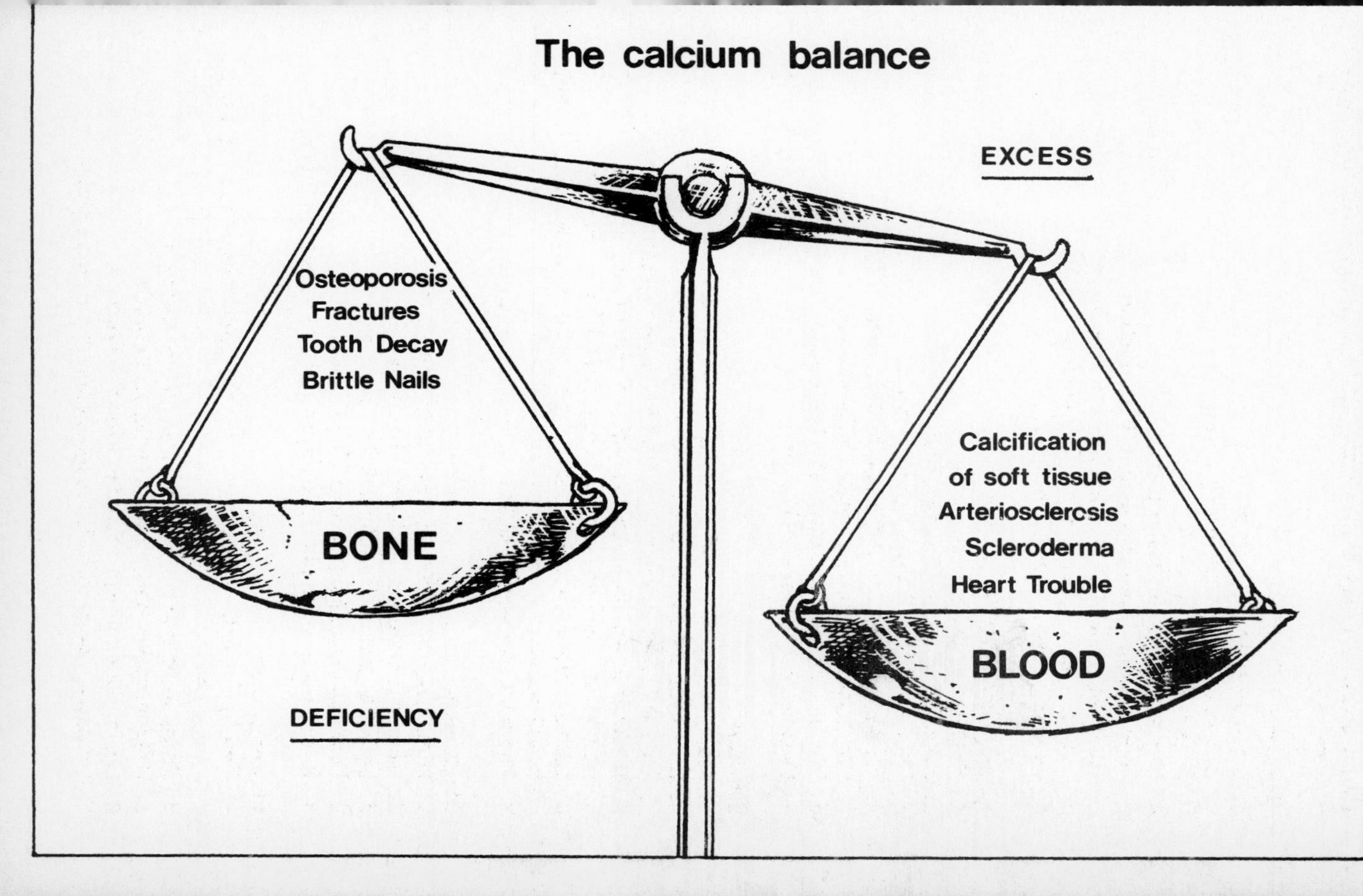
The calcium balance
EXCESS
Osteoporosis
Fractures
Tooth Decay
Brittle Nails
BONE
DEFICIENCY
Calcification
of soft tissue
Arteriosclercsis
Scleroderma
Heart Trouble
BLOOD

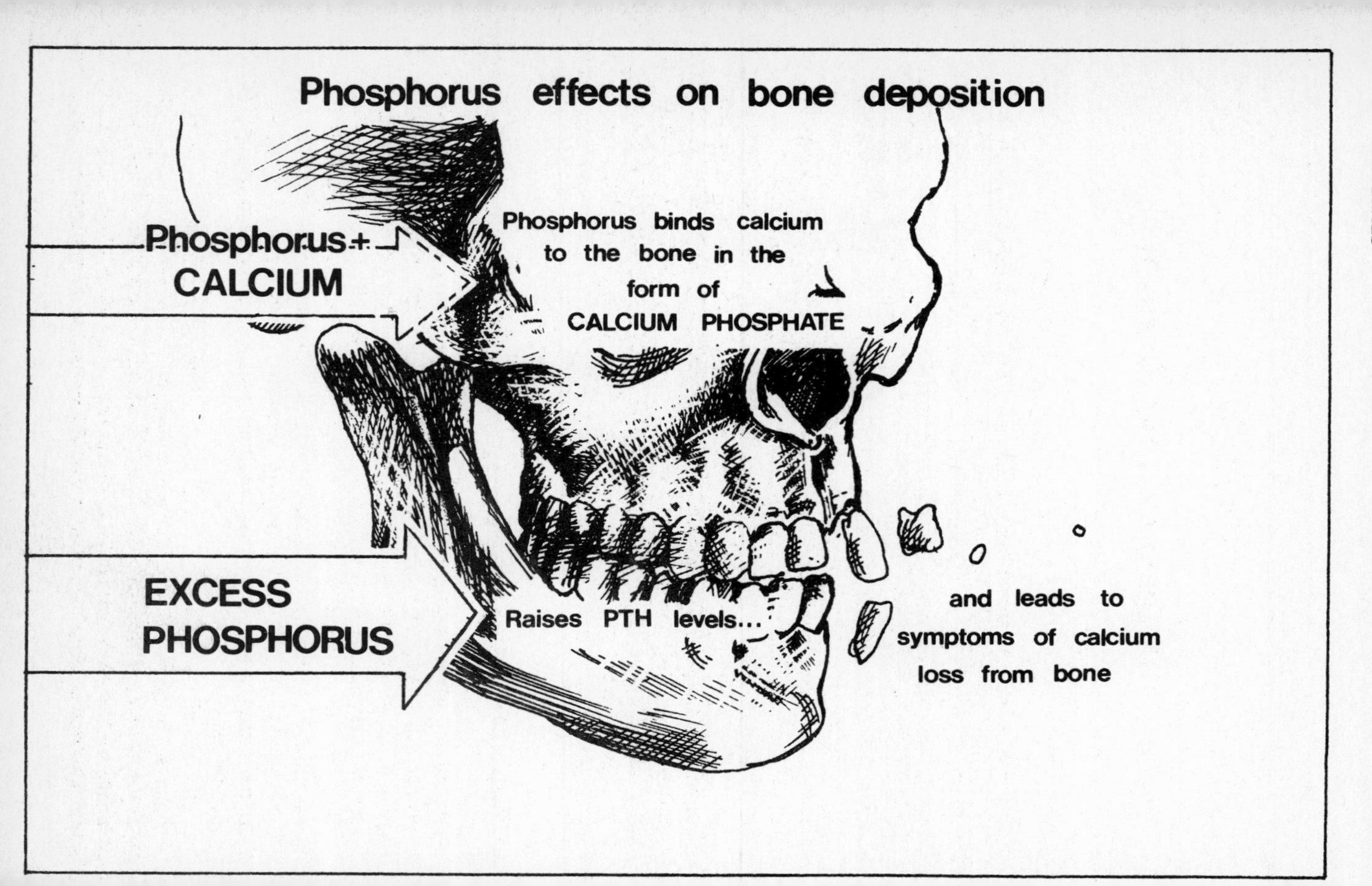
Phosphorus effects on bone deposition
Phosphorus + CALCIUM
Phosphorus binds calcium to the bone in the form of CALCIUM PHOSPHATE
EXCESS PHOSPHORUS
Raises PTH levels...
and leads to symptoms of calcium loss from bone

# CHAPTER 7

# Potassium and Sodium

Foremost among their many functions the first three minerals we looked at – calcium, magnesium and phosphorus – are all vitally important for maintaining the wellbeing of your bones. When their levels in the body are healthily balanced each works as part of a single, interrelated mechanism to ensure that the skeleton remains strong, resilient and, above all, hard. We've seen how this ostensibly unchanging, rocklike hardness depends on the constant, tidal replacement of old nutrients for new. Because of this the most static-seeming of all the body's components is in a constant state of motion.

The body is full of such paradoxes. Perhaps the greatest paradox of all is that while our bodies are strong, dense and resistant, they are composed largely of a substance whose physical properties could hardly have less in common with bone: water. Water is the single most important feature of every living thing. And more than anything else it is regulated by the two minerals we'll look at in this chapter – potassium and sodium.

## Water, Water Everywhere

An adult body weighing 11 stone contains approximately 9½ gallons of water which works out at a little over 100 lbs or two thirds of overall weight. Sixty per cent of this water is contained inside the cells. The rest is outside, surrounding and bathing the cell wall, circulating in the body as blood plasma, and collecting in the bladder as urine. It is essential that the ratio stays close to this 60 per cent inside: 40 per cent outside split as fluctuations will lead to water retention in, or dehydration of the cell, either of which can easily cause serious health problems.

If the cell wall was literally that – an impenetrable, impermeable barrier – nothing would be easier than maintaining exactly the desired amount of water inside the cell, while at the same time blocking the entry of any more water than is needed. However, 'cell wall' is a misleading, highly inaccurate term. For this 'wall' is in fact a highly complicated valve mechanism whose job it is to allow nutrient-carrying fluids to cross from the blood into the cell. These nutrients include fatty acids and sugars to provide energy, amino acids and vitamins for growth and, of course, minerals to act as co-factors in all the cell reactions. Because many thousands of reactions are continually taking place, the cell must be resupplied constantly with all the nutrients it needs and at the same time be able to dispose of the waste products from its reactions such as urea. This means that water has to pass constantly through the cells. And compared with this passage, the high pressure pumping of blood around the circulatory system is positively leisurely. For, as Gar Hildenbrand of the Gerson Research Institute in America has found, in a single second the amount of water that surges through the cell is equal to a staggering one hundred times the volume of the cell itself!

The two minerals that maintain osmosis – the 'dynamic equilibrium' of flow which ensures that the water entering the cell doesn't exceed the water leaving, or vice versa – are the ionic forms of potassium and sodium. Potassium is concentrated in the fluids inside the cell wall, sodium in the fluids outside, and working together they maintain the functions of almost every cell in the body. Each time the body has to use a nerve or muscle, the balance of the mineral concentrations between inside and out is altered. Potassium is ejected from the cell and the change in ionic balance sparks an electrical impulse causing the cell to react. It does so either by conducting a brain impulse, if it is a nerve cell, or contracting if it is a muscle cell. Once the reaction has occurred, the original cellular balance between potassium and sodium is restored and the nerve or muscle will relax (potassium's relaxing effect inside the cell is similar to the effect that magnesium has on the cell outside). This sodium-potassium seesaw action is one of the most important balancing acts in the body – more important, even, than the balance between calcium and magnesium. These days, however, the intracellular ratio between potassium and sodium is under an ever-increasing threat from many areas including, predictability, our choices of diet. In this chapter we'll look at these two minerals at work, examine the consequences of imbalances, and see what we can do to set things right.

## Potassium

Your body contains about 150 grammes of potassium, most of which is concentrated in the muscle cells. Potassium is a vital co-factor in enzymes that trigger muscle contraction and coordination, and deficiencies may cause weakness and loss of muscle tone. As we age, our potassium levels drop substantially and this is one of the main reasons for the frailty and decline in strength of the elderly. Potassium helps to convert glucose into energy and, as it raises the alkaline content in the cell, it is also important in maintaining your body's acid/alkaline balance.

The concentration of potassium in the water inside the cell is 30 times greater than that outside. Outside, the concentration of sodium molecules exceeds potassium by 28 to 1. The fact that sodium does not enter the cell and balance its concentration is a phenomenon which scientists are unable to explain as no other mineral has such trouble crossing the cell wall. In fact, in laboratory tests, sodium crosses a semipermeable membrane just as easily as any element. One easily performed experiment uses a glass jar which is divided into two compartments by an artificial membrane. One compartment is then half-filled with salt water, the other with salt-free water. Over a period of time the level in the salt water compartment rises, and the pure water drops, as water is drawn through the membrane by the attraction of salt ions. So what prevents sodium from entering the cell of an organism to balance its concentration? Scientists have long held to the idea of a 'sodium pump' – an abstruse mechanism in the cell wall that pumps sodium out whilst admitting other minerals – to excuse what they couldn't explain. This concept is now being treated with increasing scepticism, especially as biologists calculate that it would take more energy to maintain such a pump than the cell actually possesses.

Whatever accounts for this unexplained difference in concentration between the two minerals inside the cell and out, it is vital for maintaining efficient nerve and muscle function. When the relative concentrations are altered the resulting imbalance leads to a loss of well being. For example, victims of high blood pressure who suffer from excess fluid retention are often prescribed diuretics – medicines which cause a loss of water from the cells – to counteract their symptoms. But when the volume of water inside the cells is reduced in this way the body's potassium levels fall with it. On the other hand, the level of sodium, since it is present mainly outside the cell, stays pretty much unchanged. Other causes of potassium loss include pre-menstrual syndrome, oral contraception, stress, heart disease, laxatives and gastrointestinal disorders. And symptoms of this loss include weakened muscles and loss of tone; depression and mental confusion; poor reflexes; bloated sensations; dry skin; and bone and joint pain. In very severe cases victims of potassium deficiency have been known to suffer from erratic heart function and, ultimately, heart attacks.

## Losing the Balance

In each chapter we've seen how health disorders stem not only from the lack of a single mineral but also from the way in which this deficiency unbalances the overall relationship of one mineral with another. The consequences of potassium loss are no exception because the symptoms we just looked at are caused as much by an increase in the levels of sodium in relation to the declining potassium as they are by a straightforward decline in potassium. To understand how this particular balance works we have to look at the way in which the body absorbs these two minerals.

Because potassium maintains such an intimate, not to say uneasy, biochemical relationship with sodium, any fluctuations in the body level of one of these minerals is bound to affect the level of the other. This is complicated by the widespread changes in our eating habits. Potassium occurs abundantly in nature and it is present in most unprocessed foods. Since large amounts of potassium have been freely available to it since the dawn of its existence the human body has had no need to evolve a biochemical mechanism for storing it. On the other hand, ever since our primordial ancestors emerged from the sea, natural sources of sodium have always been relatively scarce. In natural foods there is a fraction of the amount of sodium that there is of potassium. As there has never been any assurance of a regular supply of sodium the body has compensated by evolving a stringently efficient mechanism for preserving the sodium it does take in.

Nowadays, however, with such a large proportion of our diets consisting of processed foods, the dietary ratio in potassium's favour has been dramatically reversed. Although potassium is plentiful in fresh fruit and vegetables, canning or freezing these goods causes the potassium content to dwindle almost to nothing. This is largely due to the fact that potassium is one of the most easily soluble of all minerals and tends to leach out of the food in the water that surrounds it when it is frozen or canned.

The amount of sodium in foods, on the other hand, is increasing all the time. This has nothing to do with that small amount of sodium that occurs naturally in food and everything to do with the additives that manufacturers use to adulterate their products. Many different forms of sodium are added to processed food. They include: sodium nitrate, which is often added as a preservative to processed meats such as bacon and sausages; monosodium glutamate, a substance that appears in the ingredients list on tins and packets with the ubiquity of seagulls on a rubbish tip, and is employed as a 'flavour enhancer'; sodium bicarbonate, added to the ingredients of cakes to make them rise when cooked; sodium citrate, often used in powdered foods as an acidity regulator; and sodium benzoate, which is added to children's soft drinks such as squashes. Of course, the most commonly used form of sodium is sodium chloride, or common table salt, which as well as occurring regularly in processed food is liberally sprinkled on our meals.

Although we now eat many times the quantity of sodium that our ancestors did our bodies still behave as if sodium were a rare and treasured commodity. Hence, almost all the sodium we eat is hoarded. Potassium, on the other hand, is so plentiful that the body will happily excrete large amounts if the conditions dictate. Today we have reached a situation where the body is absorbing more and more sodium. Conversely, a host of factors which range from the losses incurred by food processing to stress and the widespread use of certain diuretics and laxatives are causing our potassium levels to plummet.

What happens when the sodium to potassium ratio rises in sodium's favour? First, the flow of nutrients into the cell, and thus every aspect of cell metabolism, is interfered with. This means that the manufacture of proteins will decline and with it the cell's ability to repair itself and generate protein for new structures. This is why a loss of potassium can lead to dry, flaky skin. It may also be one of the contributing factors in joint pains. For each joint head, despite the soft, spongy cushions of synovial fluid that separate it from an opposing socket or hinge, is subjected to enormous physical stresses which cause a lot of wear and tear. As a result their cells must be repaired at a much faster rate than many other parts of the body. Potassium loss slows this repair rate down and can lead to a deterioration of the joints similar to arthritis.

The second crucial aspect of cell metabolism to be affected is energy production. Basically there are two major means of energy release in the body: one from glycogen, the other from fat. Glycogen is metabolized from blood sugar and is stored, ready for use, as carbohydrate. In this form energy can be summoned instantaneously to help the body respond to its immediate needs, providing the fuel for strenuous activities. Athletes tend to eat a lot of glucose, a good source of blood sugar, prior to heavy bouts of training or competition to give them an almost explosive release of energy, and it is a tradition among marathon runners to eat a large meal of pasta on the night preceding their run in order to build up their supplies of carbohydrates. The energy made available to the body from fat, on the other hand, takes very much longer to come into effect. The two different fuel sources therefore meet two different requirements – glycogen for immediate strength, fat for longer-term stamina. The body obviously needs both. Yet without potassium its supplies of glycogen will be cut dramatically. Why is this?

Potassium is an enzyme co-factor in the conversion of blood sugar to glycogen. Without it the blood sugar will circulate unconverted while existing supplies of glycogen will dwindle. Blood sugar is itself a fuel but comparing its energy value with that of glycogen is like comparing a stack of tinderwood with a yule log. Therefore, if the body is active, the blood sugar will be consumed rapidly, leading to an immediate, sometimes distressing, fall-off of energy and a feeling of fatigue, languor and a loss of elasticity in the muscles when exercise is attempted. If, on the other hand, the body is not active, the excess, unconsumed blood sugar will trigger a release of insulin – a hormone whose job it is to monitor and regulate blood sugar levels – causing the blood sugar to be stored as fat. This may even lead to low blood sugar levels also known as hypoglycemia.

More important even than a decline in protein metabolism, or energy loss, or low blood sugar are the consequences of the changes in water pressure inside the cell that occur when potassium is lost. As we've seen, the osmotic balance between potassium and sodium is a vital contributing factor in determining the actions of nerve and muscle cells. An increase in the relative levels of sodium in the cells will cause water retention as the cell draws in fluid from outside to reduce the concentration. The damage which this can trigger may, in extreme circumstances, prove deadly. Higher than average sodium in the cells, for example, is recognized as a common cause of hypertension. Don't forget that as potassium is responsible – with magnesium – for relaxing muscles after contraction a loss of potassium will encourage the heart to beat harder and more erratically and the arms and legs to cramp easily. Combined with the sodium-related hypertension this can lead to fibrillation, arteriosclerosis and heart attack. And we've already seen how diuretics prescribed to reduce the blood pressure cause the kidneys to excrete even more potassium and so aggravate the overall problem.

In a recent study at the university of Pittsburgh using 2000 volunteers, doctors found that those of the group with normal blood pressure all ate diets which were lower in sodium and higher in potassium than those with high blood pressure. As a corollary to this, they realized that low blood pressure doesn't just depend on reducing the amount of sodium eaten – which is the popularly held belief – it also requires an increase in the potassium intake.

On average, people who eat processed foods ingest around 10 grammes of sodium a day in one form or another, whereas their potassium intake often drops to less than a gramme. Dramatic changes in hypertension have been observed when the sodium intake is cut to no more than 3 grammes and the potassium raised to match it. In fact some nutritionists feel that even greater advances would be made by increasing the potassium intake further, to fully double that of the sodium. This isn't a very difficult thing to do. In essence it means cutting down the amount of processed food in your diet – better still, eradicating it completely – and experimenting with other flavourings in the food you prepare for yourself such as spices, herbs, live yoghurt or whatever takes your fancy. If you do decide to use salt, your best bet is sea salt, which is high in most of the minerals, rather than ordinary salt which only contains sodium and chloride. Finally, eat lots of fresh fruit and vegetables.

## In defence of sodium

Having spent most of this chapter painting a picture of sodium as a dietary mischief maker, it is worth pointing out that while we certainly eat too much of it, it is a very important mineral. There are approximately 100 grammes of sodium in the body, a third of which is packed into the bone. A small fraction of the remainder combines with other minerals in the blood to prevent them from clogging. The rest, as we know, is found in the fluid surrounding the cells, helping to regulate the passage of nutrients, transmissions of nerve impulses, muscle tone and fluid volume.

We've seen how excess sodium increases the fluid volume inside the cells. On the other hand, a decline in the levels of sodium in the body causes more water to leave the cells than enters and, in time, results in dehydration. Normally, since sodium is present in such large amounts, a sodium loss of this nature would be very unlikely. However, in some circumstances it is quite common. Diarrhoea makes the body lose sodium. So does sweating. Intense physical activity in hot weather can make people lose up to 8 grammes of sodium in a day. This leads to problems which are as familiar to long-distance runners as they are to miners: nausea, vomiting, dizziness, cramp, exhaustion, apathy, and even circulatory problems. However, rather than simply taking extra salt to compensate, it is in fact more important to replace the lost water as it is this which re-establishes the cellular equilibrium. The same principle holds true when you eat a meal with a lot of salt – you become thirsty as your body attempts to dilute the higher than normal concentrations of salt.

## At-a-glance Guide to Potassium and Sodium

### *A. Potassium Metabolism*

| Potassium: | Potassium deficiency: |
|---|---|
| Converts blood sugar to glycogen for efficient energy storage and release | Causes loss of energy; fatigue; languor; low blood sugar |

| | |
|---|---|
| Relaxes nerves and muscles after contraction. Keeps heart rhythms normal | Causes cramp; loss of elasticity in muscles; harder, more erratic heartbeat; angina; arteriosclerosis; heart attack |
| Helps to regulate the body's water balance | Leads to water retention; high blood pressure |
| Aids efficient cell metabolism, encouraging growth and reproduction | Leads to loss of skin elasticity; dandruff; skin complaints; joint pains; degenerative bone diseases |

*Sodium*

| Sodium: | Sodium excess: |
|---|---|
| Helps to regulate the body's water balance | Causes high blood pressure; nausea; cramp; vomiting; dizziness; exhaustion |
| With potassium it helps to control nerve and muscle function | Causes irregular heartbeat; cramp; loss of muscle strength |

*Potassium content of food in milligrammes per 100 grammes*

Kelp 3292
Brewers' yeast 1700
Raisins 763
Peanuts 674
Dates 648
Avocados 604
Spinach 470
Mushrooms 414
Salmon 410
Potatoes 407
Brussel Sprouts 390
Broccoli 382
Liver 380
Bananas 370
Carrots 341
Kidneys 310
Cauliflower 295
Sweetcorn 280
Asparagus 278
Melon 250
Chicken 250
Tomatoes 244
Brown rice 214
Peaches 202
Oranges 200
Mangos 189
Lobster 180
Strawberries 164
Grapes 158
Milk 140
Apples 110
Eggs 100

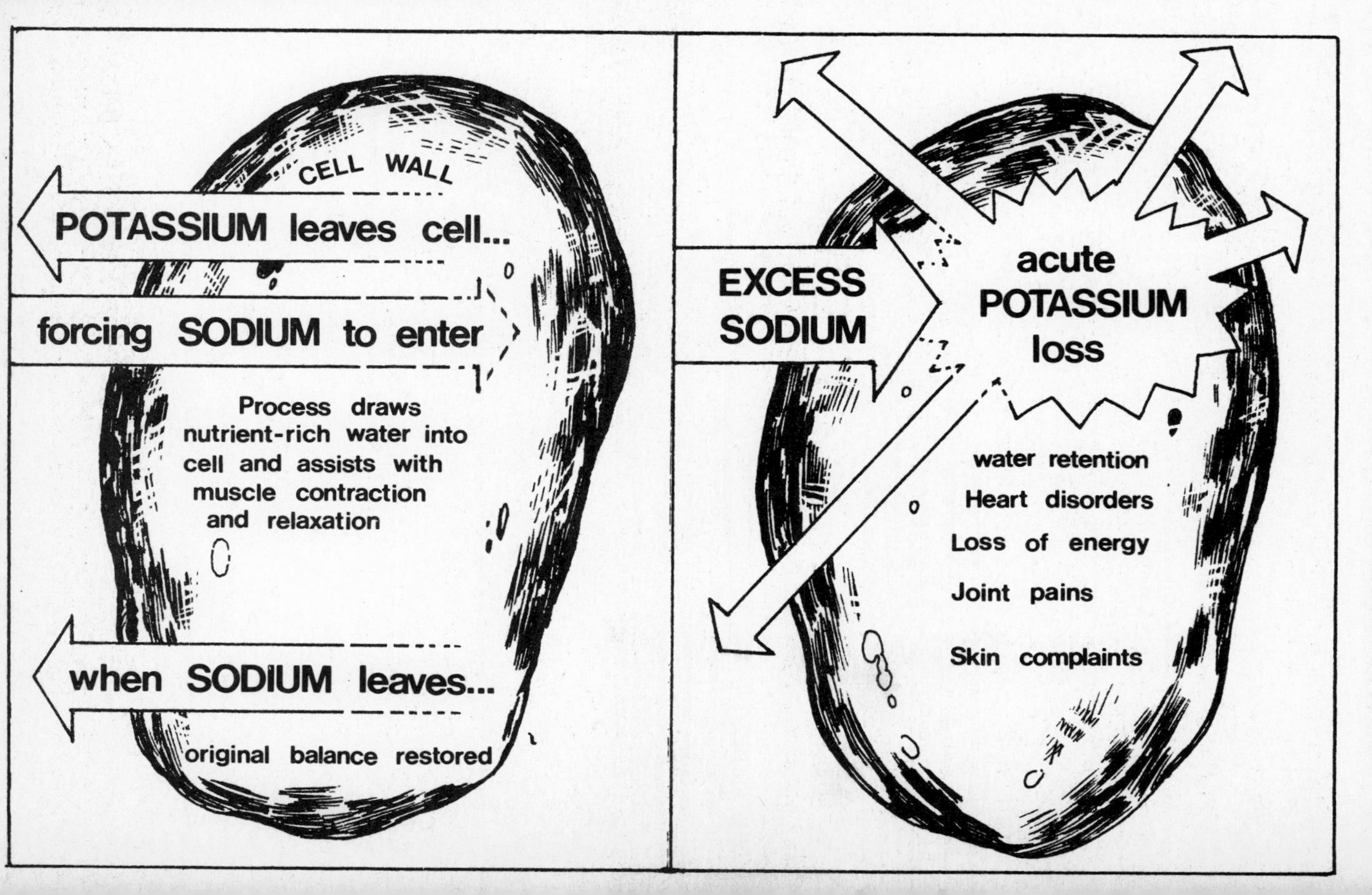
CELL WALL
POTASSIUM leaves cell...
forcing SODIUM to enter
Process draws nutrient-rich water into cell and assists with muscle contraction and relaxation
when SODIUM leaves...
original balance restored
EXCESS SODIUM
acute POTASSIUM loss
water retention
Heart disorders
Loss of energy
Joint pains
Skin complaints

*Sodium content of food in milligrammes per 100 grammes*

Kelp 3007
Green olives 2400
Cheddar cheese 700
Cottage cheese 229
Lobster 210
Celery 126
Eggs 122
Cod 110
Spinach 71
Lamb 70
Pork 65
Chicken 64
Beef 60
Milk 50
Turnips 49
Carrots 47
Yoghurt 47
Lentils 30
Raisins 27
Broccoli 15
Mushrooms 15
Onion 10
Brown rice 9
Avocados 4
Tomatoes 3

# PART THREE

# TRACE ELEMENTS

CHAPTER 8

# Iron, Copper and Zinc

Since the body contains large amounts of each macro-mineral, it is not surprising to find that they influence each other's metabolism so closely. It is rather like the same four or five people repeatedly, and unavoidably, bumping into each other as they mix at a small party. In fact, calcium, magnesium and phosphorus relate so closely that it is sometimes impossible to think of them as separate elements.

In contrast you would think that trace elements, as they are present in the body in sometimes immeasurably small amounts, would have little bearing on each other. After all, with the change in scale, this would be like our party-goers expecting to bump into each other while circulating in a throng of half a million people during the Pope's blessing in St Mark's Square. And yet, in biochemical terms, this is exactly what happens all the time. The relationships between these minutely occurring minerals are no less important than those between the macro-minerals. That's why, in the next four chapters, we'll be looking at the trace minerals in small, closely related groups, starting with iron, copper, and zinc.

Although these minerals are measured in tiny fractions compared to some of the macro-minerals, the roles they perform are equally important, though they do not contribute greatly to the body's major structural requirements such as forming bone and muscle, or have much influence on the massive hydrostatic forces in the body which control nerve and muscle action. Let's look at these minerals at work in the body, both individually and as part of the overall nutritional mechanism.

## Iron

When we think of iron we tend to imagine a hard, implacable, resistant metal. After all, some of the world's most imposing pieces of architecture and engineering, from the Eiffel Tower to the Forth Bridge are made from iron. Yet, at the same time, these monuments of durability must be constantly guarded against the damage of rusting.

Although the iron in these structures provides them with great strength, it is at greater risk from corrosion and decay than any other mineral. This seeming paradox holds true in the body as well. For while iron is one of the body's most important minerals, the body is also very sensitive to, and at risk from, iron deficiency.

Perhaps 20 per cent of the population of Britain are iron deficient at this moment. And while iron depletion is greatest in vulnerable groups such as pregnant or menstruating women, people recuperating from operations and those with poor digestion, it is fair to say that iron deficiency spreads itself out over a wide cross-section of the public. Iron deficiency is one of the principle causes of anaemia. Whilst other dietary factors, such as a shortage of vitamins B6 and B12, folic acid and copper, also contribute to anaemia, biologists consider iron to be the greatest offender. The problem is so great that the Department of Agriculture, Fisheries and Food has designated a recommended daily allowance for iron of 12 mg for adults and 15 mg for pregnant women. That such a conservative and cautious body has recognized the need to make this sort of recommendation is a sign of their concern, and of the importance of iron in our diets. Indeed, almost half the prescriptions written each year by general practitioners are for iron supplements. So what does iron do?

Simply, iron helps the body to make full use of its oxygen, both transporting it to where it is needed and then ensuring that it is utilized properly. There are between 3 and 4 grammes of iron in the body (a level teaspoon's worth) and more than half of this is used in the blood as a substance called haemoglobin. This chemical is manufactured in the bone marrow and is responsible in turn for the formation of red blood cells, or red corpuscles. Red corpuscles are the part of the blood which carries oxygen from the lungs to every cell of the body. Half of the remaining iron is employed in forming enzymes called cytochromes which enable the cells to use oxygen in their metabolic pathways. The iron that is left over after these needs have been met is then stored in the marrow, liver and spleen.

## Iron loss symptoms

Iron depletion will reduce the production of haemoglobin and of the enzymes that transfer oxygen from the blood to the cells. With less haemoglobin to distribute the oxygen from the lungs and fewer enzymes to make it available for cellular activity, oxygen starvation will result. This in turn will lead to a general decline in efficiency of the cells. Oxygen provides the basis of life. Nothing can be compared to the damage that oxygen starvation causes. Often one of the first experiments that schoolchildren are shown uses a burning candlestick standing in a centimetre of water. A glass cylinder is then placed over the candle with its rim in the water to prevent air from entering. The candle burns up the oxygen in the cylinder, then flickers, splutters and dies. This simple experiment is the most graphic possible demonstration of the need for oxygen.

An oxygen environment allows the candle to burn and release the energy contained in the wick and the wax, and it is also oxygen that provides the fuel for the chemical reactions which enable the body to live – in fact, *are* the human body's life. Iron deficiency will literally suffocate the body in the same way that the sealed cylinder snuffs out the candle. Every metabolic pathway – from the creation of ribosomes for growth and reproduction, and enzymes for glucose metabolism and energy production, to muscular contraction and thought – need oxygen. Therefore, as the oxygen drops, these reactions will be carried out increasingly less efficiently. As a result less energy will be released for helping the cells to respond to the demands and dangers of living: protein metabolism will be scaled down and the hormonal secretions necessary for coping with stress, repairing damaged or dead tissue and resisting infection and disease will all diminish.

Iron deficiency is sometimes revealed by skin pallor, as the corpuscle count declines, and the loss of the red fan from the fingernails. In the membranous undersides of the eyelids, paleness may replace the customary healthy pink. The physical symptoms of deficiency range from lassitude and fatigue to listlessness and migraine. A victim will find exercise tiring and their muscles will become flaccid thanks to a loss of myoglobin, an iron-dependent protein which stores oxygen in the muscles ready to burn glucose for instant energy release. As every organ depends upon oxygen, iron loss will affect the heart, lungs, liver, kidneys and skin, leading to more serious problems such as breathlessness, difficulty swallowing, palpitations after physical exertion – sometimes agonizing – poor vision, insomnia, cramping and profound depression. A common symptom among iron-deficient expectant mothers is pruritis, an illness where the skin becomes itchy and inflamed, particularly along the soft undersides of the arms and legs, as well as the stomach and genitals.

## Iron in the Diet

Each of the 20,000 billion red blood corpuscles lives for roughly 120 days, which means that we must eat sufficient iron to ensure that every red corpuscle is replaced three times a year. For many people this is just too tall an order. One of the commonest causes of iron deficiency results simply from not eating enough iron-rich foods. Despite the fact that many vegetables – particularly the green, leafy variety – contain large amounts of iron, they take the form of so-called 'non-haems': they are not readily available for absorption through the gut well. Meats and fish, on the other hand, are high in the 'haem' form of iron meaning that it is much more bio-available.

Phytic acid and oxalic acid, found in wheats and green vegetables respectively, form strong insoluble compounds with the iron. High calcium foods can aid absorption here by binding with these acids and allowing the iron an easier passage.

Experts estimate that the body is likely to absorb up to three times as much iron from a diet that includes meat than from an exclusively vegetarian diet. This is obviously a problem for vegans. Although they generally organize their diets with more insight and responsibility than most people – by including a rich assortment of soy products, leaves and pulses for their iron content – a marginal iron deficiency might be difficult to avoid, especially if they also exclude high-calcium dairy foods. They can compensate by loading their diets with exceptionally rich and bio-available iron sources such as blackstrap molasses, watercress, raisins, cinnamon and grapes, or with iron supplementations, although this is advisable only in extreme cases of iron deficiency.

## Iron Absorption and Loss

Once the iron is absorbed into our bodies, whatever isn't needed immediately is stored very effectively. Unlike most minerals whose levels are regulated by the liver, which excretes excesses in the urine, the amount of iron your body contains is determined by the amount you absorb. In fact, it is conserved so effectively that while other nutrients undergo a fairly rapid process of ingestion, use and excretion, iron may remain in your body for life or be passed from generation to generation, from mother to baby through the placenta. You may possibly have iron molecules in your blood which once belonged to a maternal great-grandmother who died before you were born.

Since the absorption and retention of iron is so efficient, and since there is no way of quickly and safely reducing the body's iron content, ingesting large amounts of iron over a short space of time might lead to iron toxicity. For if a large amount of iron is absorbed when it is not needed, with no useful function to perform it may start to break down the body's enzyme systems. The symptoms of such an overload closely resemble those of a deficiency including fatigue, breathlessness, palpitations, insomnia and depression. This is why iron supplements should only be taken when they are absolutely necessary, and why even vegans should try to obtain iron from their diets.

Women absorb iron twice as efficiently as men. You would be forgiven for thinking, therefore, that they are at greater risk from iron toxicity. In fact, women are inescapable victims of continual iron loss and their high absorption rate is only a safety mechanism to prevent them from developing iron deficiency. The fact is that the surest way to lose iron – most of which, don't forget, is found in the blood – is by bleeding. During menstruation women lose blood, and thus iron, particularly if they have naturally heavy periods or if they use an interuterine device as these tend to increase blood loss. Pregnancy, too, depletes a women's body of its iron reserves through its massive consumption of blood. The mother is, after all, producing red corpuscles for two people. In addition, the loss of blood at childbirth is often high, due to the loss of the placenta, minor incisions that may be made during the delivery, and the baby if born by caesarian section.

Many women are encouraged to take iron supplements both during pregnancy and during their periods. Some, however, find the occasional side effects, such as constipation and indigestion, hard to tolerate –especially as this discomfort will aggravate other problems like the bloated feeling of water retention and the nausea of morning sickness –and choose not to take the iron. Losing an essential mineral like this has been cited by some experts as the cause of the peculiar phenomenon of women developing a craving to eat soil. Even when the intelligent, conscious and reasoning side of a person isn't aware of the body's needs, or of any growing depletion, there is another, more instinctive, side which is. By creating what appears to be a wholly irrational craving for soil this instinctive side is attempting to make the body meet its mineral needs by directing it to the richest of all sources of minerals – the soil.

Iron loss, however, isn't only confined to pregnant and menstruating women. There is a narrow margin between healthy iron levels and iron deficiency. Since bleeding will force the body to cross that margin, you should be wary of anything which causes you to bleed. Peptic ulcers, haemorrhoids and hernias can all lead to iron deficiency.

Donating blood may do the same. Giving blood is one of the most public-spirited and useful things a person can do. But since the donor is giving freely of their time – and body – more interest should be paid to their wellbeing. In donating a pint of blood, close to 250 mg of iron are lost. On a normal diet it will take several months to restore the iron in the body to its original levels. Yet donors are given next to no information on the best ways of replenishing that lost iron. All they get is a cup of tea, a biscuit, and a quick lie down. Perhaps the blood transfusion service is worried about the anxiety that warning prospective donors of the dangers of iron loss would cause. Obviously a cup of tea is more reassuring than a lecture on oxygen starvation. But surely a talk or free pamphlet briefly explaining the benefits of raising your intake of iron-rich foods to compensate for the loss would be a more responsible way of conducting their operations.

Who else is likely to suffer from iron loss and anaemia? Slimmers who compulsively reduce their diets without considering the nutritional consequences are particularly at risk. So too are teenagers for whom a poor diet is almost *de rigueur*. At their stage of rapid growth and development – the most rapid of all excepting the first few months of their lives – their iron requirements are very high. Unfortunately they are also at the stage where they consume the largest amounts of junk foods. Overprocessed and highly refined, these foods contain much lower amounts of iron than teenagers need for healthy growth. Patients convalescing after serious illness or operations are also at risk from the scarcity of iron. So too are the elderly, particularly if they suffer from low stomach acid.

## Copper

The adult body contains between 50 and 120 mg of copper. A third of this is contained in the liver and brain and another third in the muscles. The rest circulates in other soft tissues and in the blood. Approximately 30 per cent of the copper we eat is absorbed, both by the stomach and in the upper end of the small intestine. The exact nature of copper's functions in the body is poorly understood and no one is quite sure of the extent to which it affects the body's metabolism. What is certain is that copper is a co-factor in the production of a large number of enzymes which the body uses for triggering several essential chemical reactions.

## Copper and Iron

One such enzyme, for example, is used in the bone marrow to help iron form the vital, oxygen carrying, red blood cells. This is yet another example of the system of biochemical interdependence that the body employs to metabolize its minerals. For, even if the body has ample supplies of iron, it might still fall victim to anaemia if there isn't enough copper to work as a co-factor in this enzyme. There are numerous examples of patients who have been tested and found to have a healthy iron intake, or have actually been given iron supplements, yet still continue to suffer from the classic symptoms of anaemia – pallor, lassitude, fidgeting and migraine. And in the absence of any obvious cause these symptoms are often diagnosed as neurosis. Only in the past few years have researchers realized that these problems can indeed have a physical cause – copper deficiency. Such a deficiency usually occurs during pregnancy or lactation. In fact a baby builds up its copper reserves during its first few months. This means that a mother who breast feeds is donating her copper to her child, often without increasing her own copper intake.

## Copper and Protein

Copper is also deeply involved in the manufacture of protein. It is a co-factor of an enzyme called superoxide dismutase which is, in effect, a metabolic cement. This enzyme is used to bind chains of protein molecules together into a mesh-like structure. Almost every protein structure in the body – from skin and muscle to blood vessel and (some, not all) organs – owes its flexibility and tensile strength to this cross-linking, biochemical mesh. Since copper plays an integral role in ensuring that the protein chains mesh properly, any deficiency will hinder the process. Copper deficiency results in immature cross-linking which might appear on the skin as dryness or chaffing. An excess of copper, on the other hand, by overstimulating the production of superoxide dismutase, may lead to hard, stiff skin, lacking in elasticity.

More serious than these skin complaints, however, is the problem that acute copper deficiency will lead to, especially in children. A very small number of babies are born each year with Menke's syndrome, a disease caused by a chronic inability to absorb more than a quarter of the normal amount of copper. Its most obvious symptoms are inflamed skin and tough, wiry hair. The real problems, though, are internal. The child's blood vessels – which are made from cross-linked protein – are deprived of their copper-given ability to flex, and eventually become twisted, constricted and rigid. Blood pressure builds up and the vessels rupture, causing internal haemorrhaging. Menke's syndrome can result in brain damage, seizures and, sometimes, death.

## Other Uses of Copper

Copper plays an important, though poorly understood, role in a number of other reactions, too. It is thought to be involved in the manufacture of the pigment melanin – the substance that colours skin and hair. As we've seen with Menke's syndrome, copper deficiency will lead to a loss of hair condition. This is shown graphically in the cases of animals grazing on soil which is high in molybdenum (a copper antagonist) who show pronounced changes in their coat hair, losing both tone and colour. From this, nutritionists suspect that copper is somehow intimately involved in the ageing processes of hair, of greying and whitening, as well as balding. Bearing in mind the heartache, anxiety and humiliation that these conditions cause to the easily-bruised male ego, a copper-related hair conditioner cum restorer would make its inventor a beatified millionaire overnight.

Copper is also used with some success to treat rheumatoid arthritis. Wearing copper bracelets on wrists affected with rheumatism was once laughed at by the medical establishment but today few people doubt their anti-inflammatory powers. Dr Ray Walker of the University of Newcastle in Australia conducted tests with arthritis sufferers, giving half of his volunteers imitation copper bracelets to wear, and the rest bracelets made from real copper. Even accounting for the expected placebo effects the relief given to those wearing copper bracelets was over three times the level of those wearing the imitations. Taking the tests further he found that about 13 mg of copper was lost from the bracelet a month and absorbed into the skin in the sweat.

## Copper deficiency

Copper deficiency can be traced to several major sources. The damage of Menke's syndrome usually occurs before birth and may be caused by the mother's own lack of copper (she could be the most conscientious of expectant mothers, scrupulously supplementing her iron intake, without realizing the importance of copper). Drugs, diuretics and infections all cause depletion. Then there are the antagonists. The pollutant, cadmium, prevents copper absorption very efficiently indeed. Inner cities, especially areas near factories, are relatively high in cadmium. Fluorine and molybdenum are also antagonists but the most competitive mineral of the lot – because it is the most benign – is zinc.

We'll be looking at zinc more closely later in the chapter. Basically, though, it is crucial for growth and sexual development. Since it plays such a major role in assisting growth, some women take a zinc supplement during pregnancy, not realizing that it can depress their equally important copper levels. Children who are weaned too early off their relatively copper-rich mother's milk onto relatively zinc-rich cow's milk also lose the chance to build up their copper stores. These babies may suffer from diarrhoea as a result, grow slowly, develop anaemia, and suffer from brittle, easily fractured, bones – symptoms that often disappear when the copper level is raised.

For these reasons the balance between copper and zinc should always be scrupulously monitored and maintained: if you decide to take a supplement of one, then consider taking a supplement of the other as well. This is doubly important since many of zinc's functions – like iron's – actually depend on copper. Copper is needed, for example, to help zinc develop full and balanced senses of smell and taste. Zinc is also important in guaranteeing the strength and elasticity of protein tissue, yet without copper to help with the cross-linkage its effectiveness would be severely reduced.

Perhaps about now you feel like throwing your hands up in despair as yet another facet of the metabolic complexity of the mineral balance is revealed. If zinc affects copper, and copper affects iron, then it follows that zinc too must have an indirect effect on iron. With this bewildering picture of interrelationships seeming to stretch away to the horizon it might be tempting to give up trying to improve your mineral balance at all. In fact, things are nowhere near as difficult as they seem. As long as you follow a diet rich in an entire cross-section of minerals, and balance your mineral supplements, there shouldn't be any problem at all.

Copper deficiency also leads to higher levels of cholesterol in the blood and has been linked to heart disease. Depletion has also been found to lead to bone defects and calcium loss from the bone.

## Zinc

The three roles with which zinc is most closely associated involve growth, sexual development and maintaining healthy skin. Indeed nutritionists have found that zinc deficiency is directly related to impotence, severe acne and dwarfism. As with most minerals there is no existing British recommended daily allowance although experts estimate that we need between 15 and 20 mg daily. Zinc is needed for producing insulin and to help carry the carbon dioxide in the blood to the lungs. By acting as a co-factor in the enzyme carbonic anhydrase it is also important in helping to maintain the body's acid-alkaline balance. Like other trace elements, zinc is an essential co-factor in many enzymes and probably the most important of these is one that is needed for the growth and repair of every cell in the body.

## Zinc, Growth and Repair

We saw briefly in Chapter 1 how the task of creating new protein structures for growth or repair is performed by two nucleic acids: DNA and RNA. DNA, the chromosome, is present in each cell and encoded into its twisted double helix are the blueprints for every enzyme and protein structure. This is called the genetic code. When a new structure is needed – and such demands occur hundreds of times a second in each cell – the section of DNA which contains the relevant information is selected and then bonded to a strand of RNA, also known as a ribosome. The ribosome, now an exact replica of the section it has attached itself to, then separates itself from the DNA. Now a miniature blueprint in its own right, the ribosome is used as a template by the cell to bind the relevant proteins and enzymes together in the correct order to create the desired structure, be it muscle, skin, blood vessel or nail.

One of the crucial factors in this bonding and transference procedure is the enzyme which joins the ribosome with the chromosome and allows replication to take place. This enzyme is called DNA-dependent RNA polymerase. Zinc is essential for manufacturing it. We can see from this that zinc is crucial for protein synthesis as a deficiency will hinder the replication process and in time slow down the manufacture and repair of protein.

## Zinc Loss

Symptoms of the fall in protein metabolism that zinc deficiency causes are all around us. Emphysema, the loss of elasticity in the lungs exacerbated by smoking, is a classic sign of zinc depletion. In this case the high level of copper contained in the smoke antagonizes and removes the zinc (together with vitamin C which is also important for healthy protein formation) causing the lung tissue to deteriorate and stiffen. Poor wound healing is another sign of zinc deficiency as is the appearance of white spots and bands on a person's nails. A deteriorating sense of taste and smell is another sign of zinc loss and can lead to a loss of appetite and consequent decline in weight. Not surprisingly zinc is very important during pregnancy. Newly-born victims of zinc deficiency may develop a disorder called acrodermatitis enteropathica which is characterized by large, unsightly lesions, as well as diarrhoea. It was once fatal but can now be relieved by zinc supplementation.

## Zinc and Sex

As it is an essential component of both ovaries and testes zinc plays a major role in the sexual performance of males and females. Even a marginal deficiency has been found to reduce libido. Tests have shown that zinc loss will lower testosterone in men and substantially cut their sperm count. The prostate gland is particularly badly affected by zinc loss as it contains more of the mineral than any other organ in a man's body. Dr Carl Pfeiffer, of the Brain Bio Institute in Princeton estimates that an average 15 mg of zinc is lost in a single ejaculation and since this amounts to almost all of a man's daily intake deficiency is quite common.

Taking this close relationship between sexual function and zinc levels into account, it's unsurprising that researchers have discovered that two of the three most common prostate disorders respond well to zinc therapy. One of these disorders is prostatitis, an illness which affects young men, where the gland becomes inflamed and swollen and leads to pain, difficulty in urinating and a loss of sexual ability. The other is called benign prostatic hypertrophy, a degenerative problem which affects 10 per cent of men over 40 years of age and 80 per cent of those over 80. Both problems have been treated with zinc by the nutritional expert, Dr R Bush of Chicago, who discovered in tests spanning six months that 70 per cent of his patients responded well to doses of between 50 and 150 mg of zinc. And Carl Pfeiffer has found that zinc supplements, as well as raising the male sperm count, greatly increases the intensity of orgasm. It is wrong to give the impression that zinc is a sexual wonderdrug – particularly as doing so might encourage some people to increase greatly their zinc intake at the expense of copper and iron. All the same, the importance of zinc as one of the vital components of sexual potency must be unquestioned.

## Zinc and the Skin

Skin health has also been improved by using zinc. Many victims of acne, when tested, have been found to suffer from low zinc levels. Scientists believe that zinc is a co-factor in the formation of a protein which is used to carry vitamin A – a vital nutritional requirement of the skin – from the liver into the blood. A zinc deficiency, therefore, prevents the skin from being adequately nourished and able to resist infection, eventually resulting in acne. In addition, losing vitamin A in this way might lead to boils, ulcers – both on the skin and in the lining of the mouth and throat – and body odour.

## Zinc and Immunity

Zinc depletion can also reduce a person's immunity to illness. There are several independently occurring branches of the immune system and one branch, controlled by the thymus gland in the chest, depends heavily on zinc for its efficiency and strength of response. The thymus gland fights viral, fungal and autoimmune infection by secreting the so-called T-cells – tiny organelles which are designed to combat very specific types of illness. A drop in zinc levels damages the thymus gland and may result either in a drop in production of T-cells, which would cause infection, or over-production, in which case the T-cells might actually attack the body, causing allergies and autoimmune diseases such as rheumatism.

## Zinc Deficiencies

The turnover of zinc in the body is so rapid that under certain circumstances a deficiency may arise in a day or two. In fact many people suffer from a continuing but marginal zinc deficiency with no more to show for it than white spots on their nails. Occasionally, though, things can become very much worse. Alcohol, for example, induces zinc excretion. If a pregnant woman happens to be a heavy drinker there is a good chance that her baby will be born with foetal alcohol syndrome – an illness whose symptoms include deformed features, blotchy, inflamed skin and acutely stunted growth.

As zinc is also involved in the storage and release of insulin – the hormone which regulates blood-sugar levels – diabetics often have low zinc. Researchers aren't clear whether diabetes leads to depressed zinc levels or whether it is actually the lack of zinc which contributes to the diabetes. The traces of copper in water that has been carried by copper pipes will also reduce the amount of zinc that you absorb. And the phytic acid contained in bran will prevent absorption by forming an insoluble compound with zinc. Oestrogen also affects zinc levels; the contraceptive pill causes a drop in zinc as does the high level of natural oestrogen in the body before a period.

## At-a-glance guide to Iron, Copper and Zinc

*A. Iron Metabolism*

| Iron: | Iron deficiency: |
|---|---|
| Enables the body to make full use of its oxygen. It is a vital component of haemoglobin and red corpuscles<br>Excess iron interferes with protein and enzyme metabolism and reduces effectiveness of immune system. Causes fatigue, breathlessness, palpitations, insomnia and depression | Causes oxygen starvation which results in pallor, fatigue, palpitations, poor vision, insomnia, cramps, depression and pruritis |

Causes of iron loss: low bio-availability in certain foods; childbirth; menstruation; bleeding; peptic ulcers; haemorrhoids; hernias; dieting; anorexia; processed foods; poor digestion; copper deficiency.

### *B. Copper Metabolism*

| Copper: | Copper deficiency: |
|---|---|
| Assists protein and enzyme manufacture | Causes skin complaints such as dryness and chaffing. Causes Menke's syndrome: damaged blood vessels, seizures and haemorrhaging |
| Helps iron to form red corpuscles | May lead to anaemia |
| Helps to form the pigment melanin | May cause greying, whitening, coarsening and balding of hair |
| Helps relieve rheumatism | |
| Assists in the metabolism of cholesterol | Is linked with high cholesterol levels and heart disease |
| Assists bone mineralization | Is linked with calcium loss from the bone |

Excess copper causes zinc loss
Causes of copper loss: lactation; drugs; diuretics; infection; pollution; excess zinc.

### *C. Zinc Metabolism*

| Zinc: | Zinc deficiency: |
|---|---|
| Is used as co-factor for enzyme RNA polymerase. Essential for growth, reproduction and cell health | Leads to skin disorders, loss of weight, loss of senses of taste and smell, emphysema, split nails |
| Is needed for insulin production | May cause low blood sugar |
| Carries carbon dioxide from cells to lungs | Reduces efficiency of the cell |
| Maintains acid-alkaline balance | Causes cell degeneration |
| Is essential component of prostate, ovaries and testes | Reduces libido and sperm count, causes inflammation or atrophy of prostate |
| Helps absorb vitamin A for healthy skin | Causes acne, boils, ulcers and body odour |
| Heightens immunity | Leads to allergies, autoimmune diseases, rheumatism and arthritis |

Excess zinc reduces copper levels
Causes of zinc deficiency: alcohol; excess copper; cigarette smoke; diabetes; contraceptive pill; anorexia; high phytic and oxalic acid foods.

*Approximate iron content of food in milligrammes per 100 grammes*

| | |
|---|---|
| Kelp 100 | Cauliflower 1 |
| Blackstrap molasses 16 | Cheddar cheese 1 |
| Beef liver 9 | Asparagus 1 |
| Lean beef 4 | Mushrooms 0.75 |
| Raisins 4 | Bananas 0.75 |
| Brazil nuts 3.5 | Carrots 0.75 |
| Dates 3 | Avocados 0.75 |
| Pork 3 | Potatoes 0.5 |
| Eggs 2.5 | Pineapples 0.5 |
| Lentils 2 | Nectarines 0.5 |
| Peanuts 2 | Brown rice 0.5 |
| Peas 2 | Tomatoes 0.5 |
| Chicken 1.5 | Celery 0.5 |
| Salmon 1 | Cottage cheese 0.5 |
| Broccoli 1 | Apples 0.5 |

*Approximate copper content of food in milligrammes per 100 grammes*

| | |
|---|---|
| Oysters 14 | Barley 0.4 |
| Brazil nuts 2.3 | Shrimps 0.3 |
| Almonds 1.4 | Olive oil 0.3 |
| Hazelnuts 1.3 | Carrots 0.3 |
| Walnuts 1.3 | Molasses 0.2 |
| Beef liver 1.1 | Whole wheat 0.2 |
| Lamb chops 0.7 | Chicken 0.2 |
| Butter 0.4 | Eggs 0.2 |
| Pork loin 0.4 | Turnips 0.2 |

*Approximate zinc content of food in milligrammes per 100 grammes*

| | |
|---|---|
| Steak 5.5 | Sardines 3 |
| Lamb chops 5.5 | Chicken 2.5 |
| Split chips 4 | Hazel nuts 2.5 |
| Brazil nuts 4 | Anchovies 2 |
| Beef liver 4 | Tuna 2 |
| Egg yolk 3.5 | Haddock 2 |
| Oats 3 | Shrimps 1.5 |
| Almonds 3 | Turnips 1 |

Parsley 1
Potatoes 1
Carrots 0.5
Wholewheat bread 0.5
Milk 0.5
Pork chops 0.5
Grape juice 0.5
Olive oil 0.5
Cauliflower 0.5
Spinach 0.2
Cabbage 0.2
Lentils 0.2
Butter 0.2
Cucumber 0.1

CHAPTER 9

# Iodine and Manganese

Without exception, none of the minerals we've looked at so far work on the body independently, but rather as part of an interlocking metabolic mechanism. It is the way in which each one affects the others that determines the body's level of health. For this reason, prescribing a single mineral to relieve a problem without considering the others is unlikely to meet with much success. Witness the connection between calcium, magnesium and phosphorus; potassium and sodium; and iron, copper and zinc. Each one depends for its efficient metabolism on other minerals which are closely involved in the same reactions. It is an unwritten law that no substance can effectively nourish the body without cooperating with other substances. Since laws are made with the idea that they are likely to be broken, it's time we introduced the lawbreaker of the mineral world: iodine. For, unlike any other mineral, iodine can singlehandedly influence your rate of growth, the health of your skin, your energy level and your mental development. In fact iodine is so important that it is one of the three minerals in Britain to have a recommended daily allowance (140 mcg).

The key to iodine's tremendous influence in the body lies in the thyroid gland. The body holds perhaps 40 mg of iodine and half of this is concentrated solely in this one organ. Situated at the base of your neck, the thyroid gland uses iodine to manufacture and secrete two hormones, thyroxin and tri-iodothyronine. It is their job to govern the body's basal metabolism rate – the speed at which oxygen is burned in the body to release energy for all the vital biochemical reactions that produce growth.

## Iodine Deficiency

A long-term deficiency of either of these iodine-dependent hormones will result in low vitality and energy, coarse, dry skin, lank, dry hair, low resistance to disease and obesity. Other symptoms will include loss of control of the facial muscles – which may lead to drooling – retarded development of the sexual organs, impotence and cretinism.

Perhaps the most widely recognized of all the signs of iodine deficiency is goitre. This disorder occurs when the cells of the thyroid gland, starved of iodine, swell up. As the situation worsens the victim's neck will start bulging, hindering free movement and causing breathlessness as it constricts the oesophagus. The fact that goitre was traditionally much more common in certain parts of the world than others suggested to researchers that geographical factors had a major bearing on iodine deficiency. Goitre was once very common in parts of Derbyshire (in fact, it is also called Derbyshire neck) and in the Cotswolds. Both these areas support a high level of farming and both have bedrocks of porous limestone. Scientists have since discovered that crops and livestock from areas of limestone soil tend to be iodine-deficient. Great swathes of soil across the Earth, from the Great Lakes to parts of the Ukraine, are low in iodine for this reason.

Nowadays, with highly developed transport systems, the threat of eating food which has been cultivated in low iodine areas is reduced because it is mixed up with food rich in iodine. Diets are much more varied now and where people once had to depend for their nutrition on local produce (thus concentrating the amount of iodine-deficient food they might eat) they can now obtain a wide cross-section of food from many different areas which offsets the risks.

## Iodine and goitrogens

The effects of iodine deficiency are now well understood and those living in high-risk areas can be easily protected with iodine supplements. Nonetheless, over 200 million people today still suffer from the disorders of iodine depletion and researchers are looking for other causes of deficiency. Their work has focused on a group of substances called goitrogens which prevent the thyroid gland from absorbing the all-important iodine. One such goitrogen is the mineral manganese, which works against iodine as a powerful antagonist. One of the richest sources of manganese is tea, and while the average British intake of five or six cups a day isn't likely to affect your iodine levels, drinking very much more than this almost certainly will.

Another rich source of iodine-antagonizing manganese is cabbage. Its effect on iodine is graphically demonstrated by the results of a health improvement programme conducted in Tasmania in the early sixties. At that time, nutritionists discovered an iodine deficiency in the soil and recommended giving iodine supplements to all schoolchildren. Up until then the incidence of goitre was very high and the nutritionists confidently predicted a drop as soon as the iodine was administered. Imagine their surprise when, after two years of study, it was revealed that the incidence of goitre had actually started to rise, coinciding exactly with the introduction of iodine supplementation. At first they were at a loss to explain the figures. The accepted wisdom that iodine is the most important nutrient in preventing goitre was in serious danger of being dismissed out of hand.

Then the nutritionists realized that free milk had been introduced into schools at the same time as the iodine. Clutching at whatever straw they were offered, they traced the milk back to its source. They found that the milk had been obtained from cows fed almost exclusively on kale – a form of cabbage with one of the highest manganese contents of any food. The deficiencies in the schoolchildren had been caused simply by these high levels of manganese which had antagonized the iodine. And when the manganese was removed the incidence rate of goitre started to drop.

## Iodine and pregnancy

As with most nutritional deficiencies, pregnant and lactating women are those at the greatest risk from deficiencies. If the mother becomes iodine deficient during her pregnancy her baby might be born with hyperthryroidism. It will grow slowly, have difficulty learning and be vulnerable to infection and disease. Girls passing through puberty are also at a greater risk from deficiency.

## Iodine sources

The best natural sources of iodine come from seafood such as fish and oysters, kelp and seaweed (laver bread, the Welsh delicacy, is loaded with iodine) and sea salt. This is why, before widespread transportation of food from one part of the country to another became commonplace, people living a long way inland with no access to fresh fish were much more vulnerable to iodine deficiency. However, even today, with sea produce readily available for all, we are not necessarily better off. Storage and processing often cause a drastic loss of iodine. Boiling fish, for example, is the worst possible way of preparing it since most of the iodine disappears into the water. Baking or frying are much healthier ways of cooking your fish, particularly if you keep the iodine-rich juices and use them as a condiment. Also, try to ensure that your fish is freshly caught. Many of the hauls landed by fishermen these days have spent days, weeks, or even months frozen in the trawler's hull. When the fish are landed and allowed to thaw the iodine leaches out along with the melting ice, so that even before you can start to prepare the fish it may be iodine deficient. In Japan, where freshly-caught fish – often eaten raw – is a dietary staple, iodine deficiency is almost unheard of. Even though you may not want to eat fish as often as the Japanese, including it in your meals at least once a week is highly recommended.

## Iodine and radiation

In April 1986, iodine was pushed into the world's news headlines with the explosion of a nuclear reactor at Chernobyl in Russia. The cloud of irradiated dust that was released contained high levels of radioactive iodine. Stories abounded of chemists in central and western Europe under siege from crowds clamouring for iodine pills to protect them from thyroid cancer. How was iodine supposed to help? Quite simply, iodine is very easily absorbed, mainly in the small intestine. Raising your intake will, in effect, saturate the thyroid gland with iodine and thereby reduce its iodine demands to nil. Therefore, when the particles of radioactive iodine reach the body, if there is no room left in the thyroid for them to be absorbed they will pass harmlessly through. Given the number of nuclear power stations that dot the country, and the less than totally convincing assurances of safety from our great and good, a big bottle of iodine tablets might make a good addition to your bathroom cabinet.

## Manganese

While we know exactly what iodine does in the body, what hormones it stimulates and the functions they perform, manganese presents a much more shadowy, less easily understood picture. To start with it is one of the few nutrient minerals (as opposed to toxins) not to be given an RDA by any country, for the simple reason that scientists are unable to decide how much or how little the body needs. What is certain is that the human body holds between 10 and 20 mg of manganese, most of which is stored in the bones, liver and kidneys.

## Manganese and the Body

Scientists agree that manganese plays several important but ill-defined roles in triggering a number of reactions. It is involved in energy production, bone formation, sugar and protein metabolism and muscle contraction. It helps to build the structure of the foetus in the womb. It is part of the enzyme system that helps the body to rid itself of ammonia – the poisonous by-product of protein metabolism – by forming urea. Manganese also contributes to fertility, brain function and inner ear balance. Since it is involved in muscle contraction doctors sometimes diagnose heart attacks from higher than normal levels of manganese in the blood, and therefore lower than normal in the muscles. Manganese loss might lead to convulsions, skipped heartbeat, weight loss, skin complaints and raised blood sugar.

Since manganese is so poorly understood, researchers often try to judge its importance to the body by extracting it from an animal's food and recording the results. For example, the nutritionist, Richard Passwater, has found that manganese deficiency will lead to abnormal bone and cartilage growth as well as a degeneration of the discs that separate and cushion the vertebrae. And animals which are exposed to a manganese deficiency in the soil become lame and suffer from crooked, twisted limbs, while the growth of young animals can become severely retarded. Manganese might therefore play a role in the prevention of degenerative bone diseases such as osteoporosis.

Some therapists have used manganese as a way of relieving schizophrenia. Carl Pfeiffer, for example, believes that in certain cases schizophrenia may be caused by higher than normal levels of copper. Since manganese displaces copper very effectively – especially when used in conjunction with zinc – Pfeiffer has given high doses of manganese to schizophrenic patients with impressive success.

## Manganese and Diabetes

Without doubt, though, manganese's most important work in the body involves the metabolism of carbohydrates. Manganese helps the pancreas to store the sugars and starches obtained from our food in readiness for their conversion to energy. In laboratory tests, animals have been deprived of manganese, then fed large amounts of sugar. They react in exactly the same way as diabetics, people in whom the pancreas is unable to secrete enough of the sugar-regulating hormone, insulin. The blood sugar level, rising way above safety limits, and with nothing to bring it back down, causes convulsions, coma and eventual death.

A corollary to this research is that when a person's pancreas is removed because of disease, or if they happen to suffer from diabetes, doctors observe an enormous drop in the levels of manganese circulating in the victim's blood. For this reason manganese is often prescribed as part of a diabetic's therapy, although, since manganese is the most elusive of minerals, no one is really sure why it affects sugar metabolism. It might take part in the creation of insulin, it might be necessary for the growth and regeneration of the pancreas. No one knows.

What is certain is that treatment with it works. In their book

*Minerals: Kill or Cure*, Ruth Adams and Frank Murray tell of a young black South African who was admitted to hospital in a diabetic coma. Tests showed that his blood sugar levels were catastrophically high – more than ten times above the norm. Wondering how he had managed to survive for so long without insulin injections they discovered that the man had regularly drunk infusions of alfalfa tea. When they gave him the tea his blood sugar level sank to something approaching normal and when it was briefly withheld the levels began to rise again. It hardly needs saying that manganese is a major nutritional constituent of this sort of tea.

## Causes of Deficiency

As we have seen already, manganese is particularly high in green, leafy vegetables, especially cabbage (although it won't depress your iodine when consumed in normal quantities). However, if you boil or steam the cabbage in water which has picked up a high copper content from water pipes, since the two minerals are antagonists, some of the manganese will naturally be displaced. The same is true of the manganese in tea. Before taking water from the tap, therefore, it is always wise to run it for a few seconds to get rid of that small amount that has been standing in the pipe collecting copper molecules. Wholewheat and bran are very high sources of manganese, while refined flours lose up to 95 per cent in the milling process. People with wheat allergies, or those living in countries such as Mexico whose staple is corn, may also suffer a deficiency as the amount of manganese in corn is very small.

## At-a-glance Guide to Iodine and Manganese

### *A. Iodine metabolism*

| Iodine: | Iodine deficiency: |
| --- | --- |
| Manufactures in the thyroid gland thyroxin and tri-iodothyronine, the basal metabolism hormones | Leads to loss of vitality and energy, coarse skin, loss of hair condition, low resistance to disease, retarded growth, impotence, hypothyroidism, cretinism, goitre |
| Protects thyroid gland from radiation poisoning | |

Causes of deficiency: high limestone soils, food with exceptionally high manganese content, pregnancy, pollution, puberty, food processing or overcooking.

### *B. Manganese metabolism*

| Manganese: | Manganese deficiency: |
|---|---|
| Is involved in bone formation, protein metabolism and muscle contraction. Contributes to fertility, brain function and inner ear balance | Might contribute to irregular heart-beat and heart attack, weight loss, skin complaints, abnormal bone and cartilage growth, degeneration of discs and lameness |
| Displaces copper and may relieve schizophrenia | |
| Helps pancreas to store sugar | May lead to high blood sugar, convulsions and coma |

Excessively high manganese levels help to displace iodine.
Causes of deficiency: high copper levels, especially from water pipes, processed and badly cooked food.

### *Approximate iodine content of food in microgrammes (mcg) per 100 grammes*

Clams 90
Haddock 62
Halibut 46
Salmon 50
Sardines 37
Beef liver 19
Pineapple 16
Canned Tuna 16
Eggs 14
Peanuts 11
Wholewheat bread 11
Cheddar cheese 11
Pork 10
Lettuce 10
Spinach 9
Green Peppers 9
Butter 9
Milk 7

### *Approximate manganese content of food in milligrammes per 100 grammes*

Pecan nuts 3.5
Brazil nuts 2.8
Almonds 2.5
Rye 1.3
Split peas 1.3
Spinach 0.8
Oats 0.6
Rhubarb 0.5
Brussel sprouts 0.3
Carrots 0.16
Broccoli 0.15
Brown rice 0.14
Swiss cheese 0.13
Corn 0.13
Cabbage 0.11
Peaches 0.10
Butter 0.09
Eggs 0.05

CHAPTER 10

# Chromium and Selenium

Because they are measured in almost infinitesimally small amounts chromium and selenium are often called micro-nutrients. Compared to them even the trace elements like zinc and manganese seem abundant, never mind the macro-minerals such as calcium and magnesium. Yet, as we'll see, chromium and selenium are every bit as important to the body as any of their more plentiful and familiar counterparts.

## Chromium

This mineral is the perfect example of a substance that has been disregarded by the medical fraternity simply because of its scarcity in the body. Its levels are so low that scientists find it impossible to decide how much our bodies contain. Estimates vary between 150 and 500 microgrammes (a micro-gram is one millionth of a gram). Even if you plump for the highest suggested figure this would only give you a total amount of body chromium equal to a third of a pin-head. What is known is that the body absorbs only 2 or 3 per cent of the 80 mcg or so that it ingests daily. Yet, over the past thirty years, scientists have discovered that this minute amount is responsible for body reactions that are utterly out of proportion to its size. Depleting the body of just a few microgrammes of chromium will contribute to heart disease, circulatory disorders, diabetes, hypoglycemia, poor eyesight and impaired protein metabolism. Let's see why.

## Chromium and Diabetes

Chromium is concentrated – if such a word can be used to describe these tiny amounts – in the skin, fat, adrenal glands, brain and muscles. The secret of its enormous effect on the body lies in its involvement with a substance called 'glucose tolerance factor' (GTF). In fact so far as scientists can make out this is chromium's one and only function in the body. GTF is a compound made up of, in addition to chromium, vitamin B3 plus a trio of amino acids (the metabolic building blocks of protein). GTF works in tandem with the pancreatic hormone, insulin, to regulate the levels of sugar in the blood.

A certain amount of sugar must circulate in the blood at all times, ready for use by the cells as an instantly combustible, easily available source of energy. This blood sugar, or glucose, provides muscles with the energy they need for performing in short bursts of strenuous activity. This is why athletes often consume high glucose drinks such as Lucozade prior to competing.

Any superfluous blood sugar is stored by the insulin in the pancreas and liver, ready for release into the blood if the need arises. When insulin secretion becomes impaired, however, more sugar is allowed to flood through the body than the cells can possibly cope with. This leads to diabetes and all the terrible physical disorders which that entails: breakdown of the kidneys, body-wide pain, loss of sensation in the nerve endings, motor difficulties, high blood pressure, fibrillation of blood vessels (including the retina), coma and, if untreated, death. These catastrophic effects of unregulated blood sugar on the body are collectively known as glucose intolerance. While impaired pancreas function and depressed insulin secretion are usually blamed for these problems, experts now realize that another major contributor to this disorder is a loss of the chromium-based GTF.

GTF works literally by increasing the body's tolerance to blood sugar. It does this by binding itself both to the insulin molecule and to the insulin reception sites on the sugar molecules. This enhances insulin's effectiveness as a sugar regulator by increasing its ability to latch onto, pick up and store the circulating sugar. GTF also works by shielding vulnerable tissue cells from the sugar when it is sent through the body to meet a demand for energy. Therefore, when the body is chromium-deficient, GTF production declines and the efficiency of insulin in storing the sugar drops away, while the cells become vulnerable to glucose intolerance.

The first clues to chromium's role in helping to regulate blood sugar levels were uncovered in the late fifties during tests conducted on laboratory rats. The researchers, Dr Klaus Schwarz and Dr Walter Mertz, discovered that when their rats were placed on chromium-deficient diets their blood sugar levels went haywire. While the pancreas of each rat appeared perfectly healthy, suggesting that insulin was secreted normally, the rats still developed symptoms identical to diabetes.

On the strength of these experiments chromium was administered to diabetics, people who, up to that point, had been wholly dependent upon insulin injections for survival. One study found that the insulin requirements of those diabetics taking chromium dropped by two thirds in a month. Further studies confirmed the correlation between chromium and diabetes when they showed that populations whose diets were rich in chromium – in areas such as Africa and the Far East – had a much lower incidence of diabetes than western populations whose chromium levels were low. The fact that chromium greatly enhances the effects of what insulin a diabetic's pancreas does secrete must make it an excellent addition to the anti-diabetes armoury.

## Chromium and Heart Disease

Any fuel source that isn't controlled properly is dangerous. This applies to blood sugar as much as it does to nuclear power. When the mechanisms for regulating these energy sources are impaired the consequences can be catastrophic. We just saw what can happen to the body when blood sugar is allowed to run haywire. Yet blood sugar is only one of several metabolic energy sources. There is another source which we ingest as fat, or cholesterol. Following absorption it is converted to lipids (fatty acids) and if the body is unable to control them then, just as with blood sugar, serious illness is inevitable.

When the insulin-GTF mechanism works properly, and when your diet contains a healthy amount of unrefined carbohydrate (more of which later) there is little need for the energy provided by fat (although fat is vital for other functions such as lubricating your joints). Instead, the blood sugar is released in precise amounts from the pancreas and liver as and when the need arises. In the meantime, to ensure that no more fat than the body needs is circulated in the blood, GTF also acts to regulate the concentration of lipids. How does it manage this?

Distribution of cholesterol throughout the body is performed by two basic types of protein molecule. One type is called a 'low density lipoprotein' (LDL) and it is this molecule's job to distribute fat into the blood. From here it will be circulated to the cells and burnt as energy. The other type of carrier molecule is called a 'high density lipoprotein' (HDL) and, conversely, it works by carrying fats back from the blood to the liver.

In a healthy body the concentration of HDL is slightly greater than that of LDL. This ratio ensures that fat is stored away safely and only released into the blood when there is a need for additional energy to that provided by the blood sugar. In other words, HDL protects against a harmful build-up of fat in the blood vessels, fat which will, in time, cause heart disease. But what does this have to do with GTF? Quite simply, experts believe that not only will a good, high level of GTF regulate blood sugar, it will also increase the HDL-LDL ratio in HDL's favour. In other words, GTF – and by extension, chromium –

bears a major responsibility for the safe use of your body's two main sources of energy.

Remembering the damage that low GTF causes by allowing blood sugar to rocket, what effect does it have on cholesterol levels? Basically, the HDL-LDL ratio is reversed, fat is withdrawn from storage and surges into the blood. This buildup of blood cholesterol leads to the formation of fatty plaques – sludge that collects on the walls of the blood vessels constricting circulation. In time the victim will develop atherosclerosis and all of the symptoms associated with it: poor circulation, high blood pressure, angina, fibrillation, heart disease, heart attack and stroke. Doctors have long recognized that when a person develops diabetes their blood pressure rises at the same time. The metabolic bridge leading from one illness to the other now appears to be a loss of chromium.

## Chromium and Diet

In western society – Europe and North America in particular – chromium deficiency is now widespread and is thought to be one of the most important contributing factors to the high incidence of both diabetes and heart disease. This is due in no small part to the surfeit of processed and refined food. For example, all natural sugars, such as blackstrap molasses, maple syrup, honey and sugarcane, although low in chromium, are relatively high in sources of glucose tolerance factor. Including the regulating substance – GTF – in with the energy source – sugar – is nature's way of ensuring health through balance. However, as soon as these sugars are refined, the GTF levels drop through the floor. White granulated sugar, to look at the most extreme case, loses a whopping 95 per cent of its GTF when it is refined. And don't forget that the amounts of chromium found even in these unrefined foods are minute in the first place, and the body can only absorb a tiny fraction of that chromium. Refining therefore reduces the amount of chromium we may absorb almost to nil.

Furthermore, refined sugar, denuded of fibre and bulk, is passed into the blood en masse almost as soon as it is eaten. This increases the demands for GTF and insulin to regulate it, demands which the body might be unable to meet since it has been deprived of one of its main sources of chromium by refining. And so, as the blood sugar level rises, blood cholesterol level rises with it. The heart will become fatty and inefficient while the pancreas, in attempting to regulate the sugar, will become overstressed, resulting, as often happens, in diabetes.

The best source of chromium by a long shot is brewers' yeast. While it is hardly the most appetizing supplement available, weight for weight it supplies twice the amount of chromium of its nearest rival, beef, in an easily assimilable, organic form.

## Selenium

Like chromium, selenium is an essential mineral but one whose levels are sinking alarmingly in western diets. This drop is caused in part by a dependence on soil which in many regions is naturally selenium-deficient. And with the added interference of modern antagonists, such as man-made fertilizers and acid rain, leading to a blanket decline in selenium, many scientists believe that the loss of selenium from our food is contributing to a worrying increase in ill-health. Indeed, recent studies show that the rise in so-called 'modern' diseases such as rheumatism, allergies, heart disease and cancer coincide perfectly with the decline of selenium in our diets.

## Selenium and Free Radicals

There is less than 1 mg of selenium in the human body and it is concentrated in the liver, kidneys and pancreas. The recommended daily allowance in America is 125 mcg but, it almost goes without saying, there is no British equivalent. Like chromium, selenium has only one recognized function. Working with vitamin E it is used as a co-factor in a reaction that involves the amino acids cysteine, glycine and glutamic acid and produces an enzyme called glutathione peroxidase (GTP – not to be confused with GTF). Although not directly involved in the immune system this enzyme is one of the body's great protective froces. For GTP is an anti-oxidant, guarding the body against damage caused by the splendidly named 'free radicals'. If 'free-radical damage' sounds like a sabotage campaign organized by some revolutionary cadre – or, perhaps, more appropriately, cell – then you're not far wrong.

Free radicals are foreign substances which invade the body, and in doing so literally convert the host cells to their own purposes. These foreign substances can include a variety of everyday pollutants such as heavy metals and radioactivity as well as the ultra-violet rays in sunlight. They all have in common an electrically unbalanced, and therefore unstable, atom. To restore their stability they attract electrons from the atoms of host cells, in turn causing the host cells to become unstable. The chain reaction that results as the atom in the host cell then tries to attract electrons from another atom leads to irreparable cellular damage. This process of microscopic degradation is called oxidation and is responsible for the necessary process of decay in nature. Everything from rusting nails and rancid butter to decaying carcasses undergo oxidation. As one curve of the life cycle, it releases energy and nutrients for the opposing curve: rebirth and growth. Of course, when an organism is fit and healthy, oxidation is the last thing that it wants. In humans oxidation by free radicals can lead to heart disease, cancer, reduced immune function, autoimmune diseases, skin disorders and premature ageing to name but a few. This is where glutathione peroxidase comes in.

By expressly preventing oxidation, GTP guards against the decay caused by free radicals. GTP protects the red blood cells from attack and breakdown by heavy metals. And it plays a key role in the antibody-forming process of the white blood cells. It is the antibodies which, because of the free radicals, sometimes actually attack the body's own proteins as if they were foreign invaders, causing allergies and autoimmune diseases such as rheumatism. Because of this, selenium is widely used as an anti-rheumatism supplement. Furthermore, biologist Richard Passwater suggests that selenium, by raising the body's levels of GTP, may strengthen the immune system an incredible 20-fold or more. Giving selenium with a vaccine, for instance, greatly increases the number of antibodies produced by the body to fight that illness and thereby strengthens the effectiveness of the vaccine.

## Selenium and Heart Trouble

Selenium and GTP will also help to protect against high blood pressure – and the kidney damage it causes – stroke, and heart attack. People living on food grown from soil low in selenium suffer from a much higher rate of heart disease. A good example of this is a study conducted in China during the early seventies. Large areas of Chinese farmland are selenium-deficient and to see what bearing this had on the population, the authorities there selected 5000 young people at random and gave them selenium supplementation. To another 4000 they gave placebos. Up until then Keshan's disease, a heart disorder that affects the young, had been a common and ineradicable menace. Yet among those fed selenium the incidence of Keshan's disease was six times lower than in the control group. The effect of selenium was so pronounced, in fact, that the control group was quickly dissolved and everyone was given selenium. The Chinese are now giving serious consideration to the idea of adding selenium to table salt in the same way that we add iodine.

Theories vary on exactly how selenium – and thus GTP – achieve these remarkable results. One possibility is that GTP improves the efficiency of the cells' mitochondria. Since the mitochondria work like billions of minute carburettors – mixing and combusting the body's energy sources with oxygen – this releases more energy for the heart muscle and allows it to perform more strongly and more efficiently. GTP also displaces cadmium and mercury, two heavy metal toxins which are notorious for their ability to damage the protein lining of the blood vessel walls. It therefore aids circulation.

## Selenium and Cancer

Perhaps the greatest excitement, though, is being generated in the field of cancer research. There is a lot of evidence to suggest that selenium, by blocking free radical activity, might actually reduce the risk of cancer. Using mice which he had bred to develop breast cancer, Dr Gerhard Schrauzer, at the University of California in San Diego, fed a control group a diet that included selenium. Among this group there was only a 10 per cent incidence of breast cancer compared with over 80 per cent in the control group.

In New Zealand, another area naturally low in selenium, the age-old problem of intestinal cancer in sheep has been reduced by selenium supplementation.

The evidence about cancer in humans, too, is pretty conclusive. Nutritionists find that the more selenium that is consumed the less are the chances of developing cancers of the colon, pancreas, prostate, breast, lung and bladder. One American study showed that cancer was almost 20 per cent lower in high selenium areas.

## At-a-glance Guide to Chromium and Selenium

### *A. Chromium*

| Chromium: | Chromium deficiency: |
|---|---|
| Is a crucial factor in the formation of GTF, the substance that helps insulin to regulate blood sugar | May lead to diabetes and symptoms which include renal failure, pain, loss of sensation, motor disorders, high blood pressure, haemorrhaging, blindness, and coma |
| Helps to regulate cholesterol metabolism | May lead to the formation of fatty plaques, atherosclerosis, high blood pressure, angina, haemorrhaging, heart disease, heart failure and stroke |

### B. Selenium

| Selenium: | Selenium deficiency |
|---|---|
| Is a co-factor in the production of the anti-oxidant, GTP | May lead to cellular damage, reduced immune function, auto-immune diseases, skin disorders, premature ageing, heart disease and cancer |
| Protects against high blood pressure | May lead to kidney damage, stroke and heart attack |
| Might reduce the risk of cancer | |

*Chromium content of food in microgrammes per 100 grammes*

| | | | |
|---|---|---|---|
| Brewers' yeast | 112 | Green pepper | 19 |
| Beef | 57 | Eggs | 16 |
| Calves' liver | 55 | Chicken | 15 |
| Wholemeal bread | 42 | Lamb | 12 |
| Rye bread | 30 | Bananas | 10 |
| Potatoes | 24 | Spinach | 10 |

These figures show total chromium content rather than indicating the amount of active GTF present. The two are not necessarily related, as shown by the example of molasses. Although the overall chromium content is too low to be included in this table, its GTF levels, like most natural sugars are relatively high.

*Selenium content of food in microgrammes per 100 grammes*

| | | | |
|---|---|---|---|
| Butter | 146 | Steak | 34 |
| Herring | 141 | Lamb | 30 |
| Brazil nuts | 103 | Turnips | 27 |
| Wholemeal bread | 66 | Orange juice | 19 |
| Lobster | 65 | Beer | 19 |
| Shrimp | 59 | Egg yolk | 18 |
| Oats | 56 | Mushrooms | 12 |
| Crab | 51 | Chicken | 12 |
| Oysters | 49 | Radishes | 4 |
| Milk | 48 | Almonds | 2 |
| Cod | 43 | Kidney beans | 2 |
| Brown rice | 39 | Carrots | 2 |

CHAPTER 11

# Silicon, Cobalt, Molybdenum and Vanadium

These four elements constitute a group of minerals which may or may not be essential. With mineral research still very much in its infancy, and a little thin on the ground, nutritionists are understandably wary of prematurely establishing recommended daily intake guidelines. None-theless the research that has been conducted seems to suggest that all four of these minerals – particularly silicon – play important roles in human metabolism. Let's look at them one by one and discuss their potentiality.

## Silicon

Although it doubtless performs a variety of metabolic functions in lesser mammals such as rabbits and rats, scientists are not completely certain that silicon is an essential nutrient in man. The 5 mg or so that is found in the body is concentrated in the connective tissue and certain important arteries. Some researchers have suggested a link between diseases common in these parts of the body and silicon deficiency although they concede that such disorders might well be attributable to deficiencies of other nutrients, too. All the same, in 1973 a meeting of the influential group American Scientists for Experimental Biology decided that silicon was essential for good health.

What is really suprising is that there should be any question of this mineral not assuming a major role in the body's metabolism. For the surprising fact is that, apart from oxygen, silicon is the most abundant element on the planet. It comprises fully 25 per cent of the Earth's crust. Bearing in mind that life evolved by making full use of the available nutrients – in other words, in harmony with its environment – why was so little use made of silicon? The answer lies in this mineral's 'inflexible' atomic structure.

## Silicon the strong

Structurally, silicon is very similar to carbon. We saw in Chapter 1 how carbon, in effect, provides the architectural foundation of life. It is carbon that links nitrogen, hydrogen, oxygen, and sometimes sulphur together to form amino acids. It is also one of the key components of cholesterol and carbohydrate. Carbon is a resilient, adaptable atom which has the strength to bind together with each of these other substances to promote growth and regeneration, yet at the same time is able to release them from these bonds just as easily in order to facilitate the equally important process of degradation. Carbon is, in effect, like the perfect, understanding lover – strong and supportive when called upon but, equally, able to release his partner without rancour when the need arises. By comparison, silicon is a jealous, possessive brute. Admittedly, it can form bonds in much the same way as carbon, and is therefore quite able to form protein of sorts. But these bonds are much stronger, much more rigid and therefore much harder to break once they have formed. To maintain its enormous structural variety, its fluctuating dynamic breakdown of old proteins in return for new, the body needs a substance of great versatility at its core. And for all its bonding ability silicon would never provide that versatility.

In fact it would take silicon-based protein a comparative age to form in the first place, requiring an enormous expenditure of bonding energy from enzymes which were themselves formed slowly from silicon. Any damage to the body would be catastrophic as repair would take so long that the organism might die before it healed. And with silicon unwilling to release other substances from its bonds, the process of cell degradation – when worn out proteins are dismantled to produce energy, urea and possibly some raw materials for new proteins – would proceed so slowly that the overall metabolic rate of the organism would be extremely sluggish. Silicon-based organisms have long been favourites of science fiction writers but if such creatures really existed it is unlikely that they would have evolved very far. In fact to reach a stage of biological evolution comparable to our own they would need to have been evolving for many thousands of times longer than life on Earth.

## Silicon and Healing

Silicon's biochemical rigidity provides scientist with a clue to how it may be used in the body. Certainly the body's underlying need is for versatility, for substances that will allow for the spontaneous flux and change of life to occur at a suitable pace. But there are some substances in the body that demand the high degree of structural inflexibility that silicon provides. They include the calcification sites of bones, joint heads, cartilage, the chief artery (the aorta) and the windpipe (trachea). And in each of these cases silicon is much more concentrated than in the surrounding body tissues. Researchers believe that the different molecules in these structures, with their much greater need for rigidity that most of those in the body, substitute silicon for carbon at key points. Could it be that silicon works as a molecular equivalent of the reinforcing rods used in concrete?

In a recent study, Dr Klaus Schwarz and Dr Edith Carlisle of the University of Southern California at Los Angeles fed a group of young rats on a silicon-free diet. They found that, as a result, the rats suffered from retarded growth, bone deformity and underdeveloped cartilage as well as a distortion of the bone structures around their eyes. Even the sclerotic, the hard white part of the eye, deteriorated, leading eventually to blindness. Compared to these rats, a control group fed with an identical diet, with a single exception – the addition of silicon – enjoyed a growth rate between 25 and 50 per cent greater. Further, they grew up free of all the physical deformities that afflicted the test group. This seemed to prove that – in rats at least – silicon played a major role in giving these hard, structurally supportive areas of the body the rigidity they needed to function efficiently.

Another test that involved silicon centred on inducing atherosclerosis in a group of rabbits by injecting them with cholesterol. Atherosclerosis results from a buildup and subsequent hardening of fatty plaque in the blood vessel wall. In time, as the fat accumulates, the wall loses its pliability and the blood flow becomes constricted. Inevitably the blood pressure rises and the vessel wall is damaged. There may even be a haemorrhage or blood clot, either of which could prove fatal. All of this was induced in the unsuspecting rabbits when their cholesterol levels were raised. Subsequent tests analysing the silicon content of the rabbits' major blood vessels, particularly the aorta, showed that with the onset of atherosclerosis, the silicon levels in the aorta wall had dropped by up to 20 per cent. But when a second group of rabbits which had also been injected with cholesterol were given high doses of silicon as food supplements the atherosclerosis disappeared almost entirely.

Of course, animal metabolism differs greatly from our own in many important respects and it would be wrong to draw too many conclusions from these tests. However, other follow-up studies show that wherever silicon is fairly abundant the incidence of atherosclerosis is significantly below average. Alternatively, wherever atherosclerosis, and heart disease, is higher than normal, researchers have discovered much lower levels of silicon in the drinking water. From this evidence it would appear that silicon works to strengthen the aorta, giving it the sort of tensile strength that it needs to resist the stresses induced by plaque buildup. Since the silicon content of our arteries declines by half in the first forty years of our lives, a compelling argument is developing for using silicon supplementation as a means of protecting a growing elderly population from the ravages of heart disease.

## Silicon and skin

In time silicon might also find its way into the beautician's cabinet as an anti-wrinkling agent. Some researchers believe that it plays a major role in enhancing skin elasticity. Again, no one is quite sure why, but there are two theories.

### *1. Cross-linkage silicon*

Under the microscope a molecule of the skin protein, collagen, resembles a huge net. It folds back on itself and meshes with other molecules much like the branches of separate trees that grow into each other forming a single uninterrupted canopy over a road. When it is inadequately nourished, or when the bonds that help keep the collagen molecules meshed are oxidized and broken apart by free radical agents such as pollution or excessive sunlight this protein mesh starts to break apart, causing in the skin the wrinkling and coarsing effects of ageing. Because it provides such rigid bonds, however, silicon may actually work to prevent the separation of one collagen molecule from another, strengthening the skin and protecting it from damage.

### *2. Antagonist silicon*

The second theory also relates to the way that silicon protects collagen from free radical damage. Many of the worst threats to our health come from pollutants of one form or another. One of the most insidious and damaging is mercury. (We'll be looking closely at mercury in Chapter 13.) A certain amount of this heavy metal is carried in the air from factory chimneys, more is sprayed onto crops in fungicides – and eventually passed onto us when we eat the food – whilst still more accumulates in fish who are exposed to it through the shocking disposal of industrial waste into the sea. Ingesting this mercury makes us more vulnerable to a wide number of diseases including leukemia, osteoporosis and cancer. By breaking down the bonds between the collagen molecules it will also harm your skin. This is where silicon comes in for it is one of the strongest available antagonists of mercury, and helps the body to excrete it safely in the urine.

## Silicon and Arthritis

Silicon is sometimes used by food manufacturers to make their liquid products – such as slimming and high protein drinks as well as beer – flow freely and to prevent excess frothing. Scientists feel that the free-flowing, mobilizing effect that silicon has on liquid is also exploited by the body to maintain the health of its connective tissue. For silicon is concentrated in the fluid between our bone joints. Sacs of fluid, called synovial capsules, lubricate the bone heads as they swivel and hinge between each other, and also absorb the shocks and stresses of ordinary usage. Since one of the causes of arthritis is a gradual breakdown and crystallization of the synovial fluid – restricting movement and exposing the heads of the bone to damage – silicon supplementation may help to prevent this. As it also plays a role in cartilage formation, who knows, silicon may be on its way to becoming an essential weapon in the continuing battle against arthritis.

## Silicon Deficiency

As with most minerals, silicon is a victim of the wonders of modern food processing. Among the best dietary sources of silicon are wheat and cereals. Yet the milling processes which give us our breakfast cereals and fetishistically white loaves remove well over 95 per cent of the silicon content from these foods. As yet no one is certain whether silicon is a dietary essential or not. In fact, since so much of it is stolen from our food it would be more convenient for everyone if it wasn't. It is not like nature to disregard so potentially useful a substance, however, and every existing indicator suggests that we need it.

## Cobalt

Our knowledge of cobalt's role in the body is much vaguer than silicon's. Like silicon, the little we know of cobalt has been gleaned from deficiency studies in animals. Its only known function in man is to help the body use vitamin B12.

The first evidence to suggest that cobalt might affect cell metabolism was discovered in Australia in 1935. When large numbers of sheep and cattle contracted a disease whose symptoms included nervousness, loss of coordination and sensory perception, muscle wastage and anaemia, the concerned farm managers called in a team of biologists to discover the cause. At first the biologists found themselves at a complete loss since an analysis of soil and feed showed that the animals received a good supply of all those nutrients recognized at the time as essential. Then someone noticed that the soil lacked cobalt, a mineral which, since its body content was measured in terms of a few micrograms, had not been considered important. The team realized that ruminants such as cows and sheep were able to utilize the inorganic cobalt in the soil and that in doing so it contributed to the function of their nervous systems. When cobalt became deficient in the soil the animals displayed symptoms of this depletion.

Unlike ruminants, most animals, humans included, are unable to use inorganic cobalt directly. Instead it is used in organic form as a key component in the utilization and formation of vitamin B12. This vitamin is needed to help maintain a healthy nervous system. In addition, it assists with the production of red blood cells and the utilization of fats, carbohydrates and proteins. Symptoms of B12 deficiency in man, therefore, may resemble those of the farm animals in Australia – starting with a decline in the nervous system which causes loss of coordination and nervousness, then spreading to affect protein manufacture, causing muscle wastage, and finally anaemia when it interferes with the red blood cells. Since B12 is so closely linked with cobalt in man (it is the only vitamin to contain a metal and is in fact also known as cobalamin) any possible cobalt deficiency will be more than adequately remedied by taking B12 supplements.

## Molybdenum

Molybdenum is an essential trace element. The body contains approximately 9 grammes, most of which is concentrated in the liver, adrenal glands, bone and skin. It is used as a co-factor in the creation of a number of enzymes which are concerned with fat metabolism. As with most minerals, increasingly sophisticated food processing techniques and the destruction of the soil's natural vitality by pollution, pesticides and fertilizers drastically reduces molybdenum levels in our food and means that deficiency is today quite prevalent.

Molybdenum deficiency has been linked by researchers to impotence and tooth decay but the strongest evidence of its effect on the body lies in its relationship to cancer of the oesophagus. In the early seventies three clearly identified regions of the world – Curacao, the Caspian peninsula in Iran and the Transkei region of South Africa – were examined by scientists researching into molybdenum. While dietary levels of other minerals and food sources varied from region to region, the molybdenum depletion in the respective soils was the one constant. Once they had established this fact the researchers realized that any prominent health disorder common to the peoples of the three regions could reasonably be attributed to a lack of molybdenum. What they found when they ran tests on the populations were high, and rising, levels of cancer of the oesophagus, a phenomenon dramatically at odds with the world trend.

Molybdenum is also closely related to copper metabolism since the two metals compete with each other for absorption and their share of the body's enzyme systems. Australian researchers have found that giving molybdenum to animals suffering from the consequences of excessive copper intake brings immediate relief. Since copper excess is thought to be at least partly responsible for schizophrenia in future there might be a role here for molybdenum.

## Vanadium

When we look at vanadium we find ourselves looking at the farthest, most shadowy, least-explored corner of mineral research. The few studies that have been conducted into the way the body uses vanadium point to a number of possible uses. For one thing, it is an anti-oxidant so it may help to slow down the ageing process and strengthen our resistance to disease by protecting us from the ravages of free radical attack. For another, it is particularly concentrated in the teeth and those areas of the bone where mineralization takes place; therefore it may be important for growth. It is also used by the cells to help burn fat. In certain areas of South Africa, where the soil content of vanadium is the highest in the world, and where indigenous peoples obtain much of their food from what they grow themselves, heart disease is almost unheard of. Might this be due to the fat-metabolizing action of vanadium? No one is willing to say. Certain tests have shown that vanadium supplements can break down dangerous fatty plaques in human blood vessels. But even this isn't enough to confirm vanadium as an essential nutrient as the amounts used to achieve this feat greatly exceed the amount of vanadium we could ever expect to find in even the most natural, unrefined diet. Watch this space for further developments.

## At-a-glance guide to Silicon, Cobalt, Molybdenum and Vanadium

### *A. Silicon*

| Silicon: | Silicon deficiency: |
| --- | --- |
| Promotes rigidity and tensile strength for the body's hard, structural components | May lead to retarded growth, bone and cartilage deformity, blindness, arteriosclerosis, high blood pressure and haemorrhages |
| Increases skin elasticity | Leads to loss of skin elasticity |
| May work as lubricant to protect the heads of the body's joints | May restrict movement, leading to damage of the joint heads and arthritis |

Good sources of silicon include: alfalfa, unrefined wheat and cereals, cabbage, lettuce, beer, onions, dark green vegetables, kelp and milk (no figures are available).

### *B. Cobalt*

| Cobalt: | Cobalt deficiency: |
| --- | --- |
| Is a vital part of vitamin B12 | May lead to loss of coordination, nervousness, impaired protein manufacture, muscle wastage and anaemia |

Good sources of cobalt include: offal, fish, pork, oysters and dairy products. Soybeans and spirulina, a product derived from sea vegetation, are good vegetarian sources.

### *C. Molybdenum*

| Molybdenum: | Molybdenum deficiency: |
| --- | --- |
| Is a co-factor in fat metabolism | May play an anti-oxidant role in reducing cancer |
| Competes with copper for absorption | May help to prevent schizophrenia |

*D. Vanadium*

| Vanadium: | Vanadium deficiency: |
| --- | --- |
| Is an anti-oxidant | May reduce resistance to infection, and disease, and speed ageing |
| Is concentrated in areas of mineralization | May cause retardation of growth |
| Used by cells to burn fat | May cause circulatory problems |

*Food content of molybdenum measured in microgrammes per 100 grammes*

Lentils 155
Beef liver 135
Split peas 130
Cauliflower 120
Green peas 110
Brewers' yeast 109
Wheat germ 100
Spinach 100
Beef kidney 77
Brown rice 75
Oats 60
Eggs 53
Fish 40
Wholemeal bread 32
Chicken 32
Cottage cheese 31
Beef 30
Potatoes 30
Onions 25
Pork 25
Lamb 24
Green beans 21
Molasses 19
Raisins 10

*Food content for vanadium measured in microgrammes per 100 grammes*

Parsley 80
Soybeans 70
Eggs 42
Sunflower oil 40
Oats 35
Rice 26
Corn 15
Carrots 10
Cabbage 10
Tomatoes 6
Onions 5
Wholewheat 5

CHAPTER 12

# Germanium – New Kid In Town

Most of what we know about minerals – their benefits for our health, the dangers of imbalances – is due to the accumulated observation and research of an army of nutritionists, doctors and scientists. On the other hand, the work that has shown germanium to be a highly therapeutic nutrient – and, indeed, suggests that in years to come it may prove to be the most important single nutrient of all – has been carried out by one man, a Japanese scientist called Kazuhiko Asai. Thanks to him, this little-known mineral is now used in both eastern and western Europe, America and the Far East to bring relief to the victims of an astonishing variety of illnesses and disorders. In this chapter we'll be introducing you to this 'new' mineral watching it at work and explaining just why it is so effective.

## The Discovery of Germanium

Research into the properties of germanium began in the fifties but at that time no one dreamt that it could possibly have any connection with nutrition. During this period, the Japanese government, recovering with aplomb from the war, was conducting research in the field of semi-conductors. These are substances which are able to receive, conduct and transmit energy, usually in the form of electricity, with very little resistance. Silicon is the best-known semiconductor and its widespread use in the computer industry today – as part of the silicon chip – is due to its marked lack of resistance to electricity and its ability efficiently to transmit impulses. In the fifties, however, silicon was only one of several contenders for the role of semiconductor in the computer industry; another was germanium. A young metallurgist, Kazuhiko Asai, was assigned the job of analysing germanium's relative merits as well as assessing its availability in nature.

In the course of his research Asai discovered that germanium was not only abundant in nature but that its richest source was coal, the fossilized remains of our primeval forests. Carbon, of course, is coal's largest constituent since it forms the molecular backbone of every living thing, including trees. But why, Asai wondered, should coal contain germanium? The answer, he realized, was that in some way germanium – a mineral which until then had been ignored by the scientific world – was, like carbon, an essential, life-enhancing nutrient.

Subsequently, Asai discovered that germanium performed a variety of important roles in plant life, protecting plants from viruses, bacteria and moulds, strengthening their resistance to cold, accelerating growth and assisting in the essential chemical processes of photosynthesis. Even more remarkable was the fact that the best organic sources of germanium were those plants which were used by man for their curative powers. These included ginseng, comfrey, garlic and mushrooms. Could it be that the secret of their powers lay in their germanium content? As the evidence mounted Asai tried to extract germanium from these plants in order to produce a pure, concentrated germanium supplement. Creating this supplemental organic germanium was a task that would occupy him for over a decade. In the meantime he continued with his research into the mineral's properties, attempting to discover why it worked so effectively. He soon realized that the answer lay in the way it helped the body to utilize fully its oxygen.

## Germanium, Oxygen and Disease

There is a thesis, popular in many alternative health circles, which contends that all health problems can be traced to a lack of oxygen at a molecular level. Perhaps a more accurate way of describing it would be to say that all diseases result from an inability to regulate oxygen. For example, free radicals are often molecules with unbalanced and predatory oxygen atoms which scavenge electrons from nearby atoms to balance their own charges. When the neighbouring atoms lose their electrons they in turn become unbalanced and must themselves search for other electrons. This chain reaction can, in time, destroy tissue and lead to illness and degeneration. Indeed, the whole process is known as oxidation. Therefore, too much oxygen may cause as much damage as too little. This, according to Asai, was where germanium came in. For although he was sure that it could provide relief to the victims of a wide, seemingly unrelated, assortment of disabilities, the common link seemed to be that each disorder was affected by germanium's unique oxygen-regulating capability.

For example, Asai discovered that the mineral worked as a powerful free radical scavenger, acting as a metabolic barrier between the unpaired atoms of the free radicals and the surrounding, vulnerable tissue. Then, by preventing oxidation from occurring, germanium made oxygen available for other activities. For example, it increased the supply of balanced oxygen to the blood. Since many of the body's immune functions originate in the blood or rely on it for transportation, this had the effect of heightening the body's resistance to viruses such as malaria and influenza as well as mitigating the effects of autoimmune disorders such as arthritis and rheumatism. During the period in which he developed his organic germanium supplement Asai himself developed a crippling arthritic disorder. Yet as soon as he was able to self-administer a supplement of organic germanium he experienced an astonishing degree of remission. Germanium was also found to stimulate the production of interferon (the body's natural virus-resisting drug) and because of this serious consideration is now being given to its possible role in AIDS prevention.

The organic form of germanium pioneered by Asai is now available worldwide under different brand-names. There are reports of its use in cancer treatment, in relieving the symptoms of Parkinson's disease and epilepsy, and as an anti-ageing supplement. Health professionals also speak of its success in relieving gastritis, arterial disorders and even cancer.

It also appears to be an extremely effective pain-killer. The body produces its own natural opiates to deaden pain for short periods but after a while these are broken down by specially designed enzymes. Germanium blocks the action of the enzymes and thereby allows the opiates to be effective for longer.

Normally our average daily intake of germanium is about 1.5 mg, rising or falling marginally depending on the degree of refinement of the diet. However, researchers estimate that for germanium to have any therapeutic value intake must be at least 60 mg a day and as high as 240 mg. This is so far beyond the dietary range that the only way to obtain this amount of germanium is by supplementation.

# PART FOUR

# THE TOXIC ELEMENTS

CHAPTER 13

# The Toxic Triumvirate – Lead, Cadmium and Mercury

In one respect every mineral can be toxic. We've seen time and again how important the overall mineral ratio is. Optimal health depends upon the body absorbing adequate amounts of each mineral as part of an overall, balanced intake. Ingesting excessive amounts of any one mineral, and consequently unbalancing this intake, can lead to serious physical and mental illness. This is what is known as toxicity and it may occur regardless of whether the mineral that caused it is generally thought of as an essential nutrient or not. In excess, calcium, or copper, or phosphorus, or iron are all toxic, it is as simple as that.

There are certain elements, however, which have no nutritional value at all. Regardless of how little you ingest they work in your body as poisons, antagonizing the essential minerals, oxidizing and breaking down enzyme systems and killing the cells. These elements are known as the heavy metals and we'll be looking at them in this chapter to see just how dangerous they really are.

## Lead

We have Hollywood to thank for the sight of Peter Ustinov as Nero earnestly plucking at his lyre in *Quo Vadis* while the glory of Rome disappears in a conflagration, and of Malcolm MacDowell in the title role of *Caligula* appointing his horse as a senator (amongst other, more unsavoury acts). Popular culture abounds with the images of a languid Roman aristocracy, idly picking at a bowl of grapes, too jaded to show any emotion at the gory gladiatorial spectacles taking place in front of them, and this under sanction of a deranged, eyeball-rolling Caesar. You wonder how, amid all this decadence, they found the time, inclination, or inventiveness to build their marvels of engineering and industry such as roads, temples, arches and bridges, not to mention conquer most of Europe. And yet the gulf between this fictitious celluloid portrayal of the Romans and the reality of history is not so great. Many biologists now think that it was their very ingenuity which led to their decadence and the eventual downfall of Rome.

To be specific, the Romans were exceptional hydro-engineers. They constructed aquaducts across gaping ravines and steam-heated baths that still stand today. In many houses and villas they also employed remarkably complex plumbing systems to supply running water. Carrying the water to wherever it was needed in the house required metal piping that could be easily hammered and moulded into a thousand awkward shapes and corners. A metal was needed with more malleability than either iron or bronze. They chose lead. And from that moment their days were numbered. For lead is a neurotoxin, a poison that destroys many of the most important enzymes and messenger chemicals in the brain. As well as using lead in their plumbing, the Romans lined wine caskets with it and wrought eating utensils from it. The instability that took root in their ruling classes – the emotional and intellectual malaise, the neuroses and the madness – has become a stereotype now, yet it did happen. The decision-making bodies were paralysed, the armies lacked effective leadership and, over a relatively short period, the Roman empire declined into little more than a name.

However, since this isn't a history book, let's draw a contemporary parallel. In the words of Dr William Strain at Cleveland General Hospital, lead pollution is 'the greatest neurotoxin threat to all mankind. It is a damn epidemic'. In itself lead is not the most toxic of the heavy metals. Yet the threat of lead toxicity, and its damaging effects on the body, are much greater than any other toxin simply because there is so much of it in the environment.

Half a million tons of industrial lead are casually thrown into the atmosphere every year. The best way of discovering how much this is in terms of what the body should have to deal with is by analysing the lead content of ice layers in the Arctic. New ice is constantly forming on old and as it does so minute sediments of all the atmospheric particles that have settled on the ice are entombed. The more sediment that falls on the ice, the more that is entombed. In this way a cross-section of the ice reveals how the pollution of the Earth has increased over many hundreds of years. It is, in effect, the planet-wide equivalent of an individual's hair analysis. Analysis of the polar ice shows that lead increased fourfold from 1750 to 1940 and almost fivefold from then to the present day. In other words we are ingesting almost twenty times the lead of our Georgian forefathers. More disturbing still is one test which shows that since 1000 BC environmental lead has increased by 200 times. Perhaps the most telling point of all is the recent decision by a mining company to test the viability of removing the topsoil in the vicinity of London's orbital motorway, the M25. A spokesman has revealed that lead levels there are now so great that sifting lead from the soil taken from here might well justify the initial expense. Yet biologically we are essentially the same human beings as then, with identical mechanisms for coping with such toxicity. We have no right or reason to expect our bodies to be able to deal with such alarmingly high amounts. So just why is lead so dangerous?

Firstly, lead is a neurotoxin. To understand how dangerous this is we must first see how the nerves work. Each cell in the nervous system is separated from its neighbour by a space called a synapse. When a message is transmitted along the nerves a chemical is secreted into each synapse in turn to relay the message on to the next cell. These chemicals are called neurotransmitters and their composition varies depending on what sort of message is to be relayed. Neurotransmitters determine the sort of mood a person may experience, their level of excitability or relaxation, as well as helping muscles to contract and limbs to move. (Adrenalin is perhaps the most famous example of a neurotransmitter.) This is where the greatest danger of lead lies. For when lead is ingested it finds its way into the nerve cell synapses and disrupts the essential communication between the cells.

Secondly, lead is a very powerful antagonist. It prevents the body from absorbing many important elements including zinc, iron, manganese, calcium and magnesium as efficiently as it would do otherwise. Each of these minerals performs a number of vital functions. These are among the body's most indispensable minerals and the more lead that is ingested to displace them, the more impaired the body's health will become.

## Lead Poisoning Symptoms

Early signs of poisoning include headaches, fatigue, muscle pains, indigestion, muscle tremors, constipation, vertigo, anaemia and poor coordination. As the level of lead in the body increases it may result in impaired concentration and speech, declining memory and reduced intelligence. Chronic lead toxicity causes hyperactivity, retardation, senility, kidney damage and miscarriages or stillbirths. It also suppresses the immune system and has been linked with cancer. Dr Frederick Klenner says that lead activates an enzyme called hyaluronidase. This is the enzyme used by cancer cells to help them grow. It breaks down the structural proteins such as collagen which help to keep the cancer cells at bay. Lead, in other words, can help cancer to flourish.

Lead is so toxic that the body tries desperately to get rid of it in any way it can and this only aggravates the problem. Since the parts of the body in greatest danger from lead poisoning are the nerves and cells of the soft tissue, the body packs it away into the comparative safekeeping of the bones. However, even in the bone lead is far from being rendered safe. If it is unable to cause mischief in one part of the body it is fully capable of doing it in another. For, once in the bone, it hinders the bone marrow's production of red blood cells. As the amount of red blood cells declines, oxygen starvation results, leading to many of the problems that we examined in Chapter 8 such as anaemia, angina, high blood pressure and impaired healing. As lead doesn't easily degrade, accurate tests can be carried out to compare our own bone-lead content with that of our predecessors. Shockingly, the lead found in the bone of modern man is up to 2000 times greater than in our ancestors.

This process of bone storage is also why some calcium bonemeal supplements have been found to contain such dangerously high levels of lead. The animals that supply the bones for grinding into bonemeal are often subjected to high levels of the metal before they die – either from grazing on affected grass or hay or from being used for work in an industrial environment. One recent study traced a consignment of bonemeal that contained excessive lead levels back to its source. It found that the bonemeal had been obtained from a pair of dray horses which for fifteen years had delivered beer for a brewery, pulling a wagon through the fume-filled London streets.

## Lead and Civilization

Naturally, lead pollution is worst in highly urbanized and industrialized societies. Sediment dredged in Lake Erie from around Detroit, home of the American car industry, shows a twenty-fold increase of lead in that area during the last hundred years. And consider the effects of the 18 tons or so of lead that fall daily on Los Angeles. Is it a mere coincidence that recently motorists on this city's sprawling freeways have become so enraged by one another's driving that they have taken to shooting at each other? Shades of the neurotic self-destructiveness of the late Roman empire, perhaps? In contrast, a group of villagers from the foothills of the Himalayas were recently tested and found to have only 15 to 20 per cent of the lead levels of inhabitants of the average industrialized nation.

## Lead and Children

If lead is harmful to adults it is even worse for children. While adults absorb between 5 and 10 per cent of the lead they take in, children absorb between 30 and 50 per cent. And with their metabolisms in a state of fast growth and regeneration, requiring optimal supplies of all the essential nutrients, they are much more vulnerable to the effects of lead, both as an antagonist and a neurotoxin. In America, where the problem is taken much more seriously than in Britain, a recent study showed that 40 per cent of all children living in the city were victims of lead poisoning. A similar test, also in America, was conducted by Dr Elizabeth Rees using a group of 20 children. The results pointed to a direct correlation between behavioral problems such as hyperactivity and the amount of lead found when their hair was analysed.

These tests left the researchers with little doubt that lead was linked to everything from lack of mental focus and inability to concentrate on work, to hyperactivity in the classroom, aggressiveness and violence. What is even more disturbing is that this is in a country, America, whose lead-free petrol and anti-lead laws are years ahead of Europe in terms of stringency and application. No one can say with any certainty how much effect lead has on the children of urban Britain but with delinquency and juvenile crime at an all-time high it would be folly to say that the two bear no relation to each other.

## Sources of Lead

Even though the damaging effects it can have on the body are well recognized and documented, lead is still a widely used metal. Its presence in petrol has received much publicity recently. Adding lead to petrol is a cheap and easy way of raising the octane, or quality, of a fuel. The higher the octane is, the more efficiently the petrol burns in the cylinders – more power is generated and mileage is improved. It also saves the engine from a certain amount of wear and tear. Unfortunately most of this lead is then pumped into the air with the car's exhaust fumes. The ever-increasing number of cars on the road is matched by a trend among parents to carry their babies in push chairs instead of the traditional pram. In a push chair a baby is much closer to the road surface where the fumes are concentrated than in a pram. The walls and hood of a pram may offer something of a shield against the fumes.

Lead is also used in paint pigments. The history of art is littered with painters who, in the course of their careers, became mentally unhinged. This is particularly so for those who laid it on their canvasses in thick impasto with whatever implement they had – including their hands. Is it possible that the severe mental disturbances of painters such as Delacroix, Fuseli and Van Gogh, and their terrifying, though beautiful, works, can be traced to their lead-based pigments? Lead-based paints are still widely used in the building industry. There are hundreds of recorded cases of children who live on decrepit housing estates, swallowing flakes of peeling paint.

Lead is also a component of many pottery glazes. These often leach out if the utensils are used to hold acid-based foods. A surprising number of food cans still contain lead as well. Most cans nowadays are made from single sheets of aluminium pressed into shape. Others, however, mainly tin, are joined by using lead solder. Generally speaking the crimps that run around the rim of the can are lead-free but the seams that run vertically up and down the can, and are hidden by the labels, often contain lead solder.

Printers' ink has lead in it. This means that when the hundreds of tons of used newspapers periodically collected by dustmen are incinerated on council dumps clouds of lead are discharged into the air.

Few houses still retain their old lead plumbing but the same cannot be said for those water pipes underground. Like the Romans, the Victorians were superb engineers. So good, in fact, that large parts of the national infrastructure they built still remain in use today. And, once more like the Romans, they were ignorant of the dangers of lead. In many parts of Britain people are receiving water in their houses which has passed along possibly miles of century-old underground lead piping. Lead is also used in pesticides which are sprayed onto crops. This is bad enough as the lead inevitably passes from here, along the food chain, to man. But very often these pesticides are used in tobacco plantations. Therefore, even though there is no lead in the tobacco itself, a smoker is still assured of a lead lungful each time he inhales.

Anti-lead laws are gradually being introduced into Europe. By the mid 1990s all new cars will be designed to run on lead-free petrol. That's a start. Unfortunately, as lead does not degrade, what is already in the environment is what we are stuck with more or less forever. Lead is practically a toxic eco-system of its own. There is little you can do yourself to avoid lead – give up smoking of course – but there are preventative measures you can take. Basically this involves eating plenty of freshly grown food, organic if possible. Fruits and vegetables which are high in vitamins, minerals and fibre are the best natural safeguards against lead toxicity.

## Cadmium

Of all the toxins, measure for measure, cadmium is the most lethal. The only saving grace is that there is substantially less of it in the environment than other poisons. However, as the body disposes of only a small amount of what it ingests, the threat it poses to our health can only worsen as the cadmium gradually accumulates in the body. Although the body content of cadmium is only a fraction of that of lead, some researchers already believe that the damage it wreaks is more widespread and more serious. It inhibits the effectiveness of hundreds of enzymes by occupying the enzyme binding sites and prevents them from joining the body's various nutrients together in the metabolic pathways. It also antagonizes and depresses many minerals including calcium, zinc, selenium, copper and iron.

Cadmium toxicity is characterized by high blood pressure, kidney and liver damage, and reduced protein and sugar metabolism. There is a frequent correlation between deaths from high blood pressure and higher than average levels of cadmium. It can also reduce IQ.

Cadmium toxicity is also notorious for causing bone malformation and the most infamous example of this phenomenon occurred in the sixties in a small Japanese village on the Jintsu river. Over a period of several months the older women of this village inexplicably developed severe back pains. In time they became so severe that many of the women were unable to move without crying out in agony. Others carried on as best they could, moving in a timid, restricted waddle and whimpering with pain. The Japanese for 'ouch' is 'itai' and so, in the absence of any recognized cause, the debilitating back pains became known as itai itai disease. More than half of the affected women died of chronic bone breakage – their skeletons literally crumbling under their skins – before it was discovered that a cadmium mine a few miles upstream of their village was disgorging effluent into the river. As the same river water was used for irrigating the village's paddy fields and supplying its drinking water, the cadmium was quickly absorbed by its inhabitants.

From the Jintsu tragedy it was clear that excess cadmium seriously impairs the body's calcium metabolism. The overall calcium-magnesium-phosphorus balance is toppled by cadmium and the bone starts losing calcium like a breached dam will lose water. The older women in the village, already at greater risk from bone loss due to the decline in their oestrogen levels, quickly succumbed to the additional cadmium poisoning.

In fact tests show that women of all ages are more vulnerable than men to the effects of cadmium toxicity. Pregnant and lactating women run a special risk because of the extraordinary fluctuations in their hormonal levels. The solitary silver lining is that there is a protective barrier of tissue in a woman's breast that screens out nearly all the cadmium from her milk.

Smokers of both sexes and all ages are also in much greater danger from cadmium poisoning than non-smokers. Tobacco is one of the greatest sources of cadmium we are likely to encounter from day to day. And since almost 70 per cent of the cadmium it contains is inhaled it can easily lead to serious, long-term illness. For example, lung tissue contains large amounts of zinc and vitamin C, both of which give the lungs elasticity. This elasticity enhances the strength and capacity of the fragile oxygen-absorbing membranes, allowing the lungs to obtain more oxygen and in doing so to keep the blood pressure down and the body's cells healthy. Cadmium, however, antagonizes zinc and oxidizes vitamin C. In time this will make the elasticity disappear and destroy the all-important membrane tissue. The result is shallow, laboured breathing, also known as emphysema. It results in a rise in blood pressure, oxygen starvation and hardening of the artery walls. In chronic cases heart failure is only one step away. Dr Lewis of Tuft's University Medical School has found that many of his terminally ill patients whose symptoms include bronchitis and/or chronic emphysema have cadmium levels on average three times higher than normal. Non-smokers breathe in about 0.2 mcg of cadmium daily; 20-a-day smokers, on the other hand, inhale more than 16 mcg.

Environmental cadmium levels are increasing daily. Cadmium is heavily concentrated around factories and inner cities and on dumps where waste including rubber tyres, bin liners and plastic containers is burnt. The best form of defence against cadmium is fresh food and, if desired, nutritional supplements. Mineral antagonism is a two-way process and since cadmium antagonizes calcium, zinc, selenium, copper and iron, it follows that raising your intake of these minerals – always paying careful attention to the overall mineral balance – will prevent your body from absorbing so much cadmium.

## Mercury

Severe mercury toxicity causes brain damage, disorders of the nervous system, deranged behaviour and birth defects. Many of its symptoms coincide with those of lead as they include vertigo, loss of coordination and nausea. The most famous victim of mercury toxicity is that perennial party thrower, the Mad Hatter. Mercury was once used to shape felt hats and signs of mental instability were common among hatmakers when Lewis Carroll wrote *Alice in Wonderland*. Another suspected victim was Isaac Newton. Richard Passwater relates how, thanks to hair analysis of some lockets from Newton's head, two researchers, Dr P Spargo and Dr C Pounds found that at one time his body had contained mercury levels forty times above the norm. This coincided with a period in his life when he was experimenting with compounds of quicksilver (mercury) and sodium. It was at this time in his career that Newton, inexplicably, went mad. Stories abound of his irrational behaviour, his increasing reclusiveness and the sudden onset of greyness. All the available evidence points to mercury as the cause.

Mercury's inorganic form isn't considered to be dangerous because of the difficulty the body has absorbing it. However, once in the food chain – perhaps as a result of being sprayed onto the soil as a pesticide – it is converted into an easily ingested substance called methyl mercury.

This is known as organic complexing. As with cadmium, Japan furnishes an especially disturbing example of the damage that mercury can wreak. It took place between 1953 and 1960 in Minamata, a coastal region of Japan. Here the inhabitants were afflicted by a vicious neurological disorder that killed 111 and left many more seriously disabled, both physically and mentally. Scientists traced the problem to seafood that had absorbed mercury-containing effluents in Minamata bay. If we imagine that a certain amount of mercury was absorbed by every living thing in the water then the higher the life form – that is, the greater number of lower life forms it feeds on – the more concentrated the amount of organic mercury will become with each step up the food chain. By the time the food is eaten by man the concentration exceeds that in the original effluent many times over.

This progressive increase in concentration can be quite a problem since mercury is still used quite widely in agriculture to produce pesticides such as DDT. Many commercial seeds are also treated with mercury to prevent attack by soil fungi. The nutritionist, Carl Pfeiffer, tells of a labourer in New Mexico who fed grain which had been sprayed with a mercury-containing anti-fungal compound to his pigs. Not long after, one of the pigs was slaughtered to feed his family. Three family members were almost immediately struck down with derangements of the brain. One daughter lay in a coma for eight months before waking blind and dumb. Her luckier brother lay in a coma for four months before staging a slow but complete recovery. A second daughter was able to walk and talk with only the greatest difficulty.

Other sources of mercury include dental fillings, cosmetics and medicine. Natural soil erosion sends 250 tons of mercury into the sea every year. Pulp mills use mercury to prevent moulds forming on their paper while coalburning power stations pump thousands of tons of it into the air.

How long will it take people to realize the horrendous dangers posed by these poisons? Surely corrective measures will be introduced before our society simply collapses from physical and mental derangement as complete as that which devastated the Roman empire. Frankly, with vested commercial interests as strong as they are, with energy producers and farmers alike wedded to methods that continue to saturate our environment with such toxins, the future looks far from rosy.

# CHAPTER 14

# Aluminium and Arsenic

While these two elements are nowhere near as harmful as the toxic heavy metals we looked at in the last chapter, research shows that they do pose a certain threat to health. Let's see how seriously we should take that threat.

## Aluminium

Nutritionists have long agreed that aluminium is of no nutritional value to the body. It is a very light metal and at one time there was even a suggestion that the human body was unable to absorb it at all. Unfortunately, research conducted in the last twenty years has forced nutritionists to revise substantially this view. They now realize that the body not only ingests aluminium but that once it is allowed to circulate it acts like a toxin. Like lead, it may cause serious neurological damage. High traces of aluminium have been found in victims of both Alzheimer's disease and Parkinson's disease. These are illnesses which affect the nerve and motor neuron cells of the body, impairing intelligence, concentration, language and movement. While they tend to be confined to the elderly, they may affect anyone at any time of life. The incidence of Parkinson's disease, particularly, is increasing at an alarming rate among the young. Its most easily recognizable characteristic is a loss of coordination and uncontrollable shaking which, in its later stages, renders even the simplest of mechanical tasks, such as picking up a cup, impossible.

Scientists think that aluminium makes the body more vulnerable to these diseases by forcing its way into the nerve cells. Once there it clogs the nerve fibres in the brain – thereby preventing the electrical messages from being relayed efficiently to the body – and binds to the DNA of the cells to prevent effective replication and renewal of nerve cell tissue. A recent test showed that there was between ten and thirty times more aluminium in the nerve cells of Parkinson's disease victims than the average. And Dr Don Crapper of the University of Toronto has calculated that there is at least four times as much aluminium as is normal in the cells of senility patients. It has also been closely linked with hyperactivity in children.

Aluminium also adversely affects the hormonal process which stores calcium in the bone. When the levels of aluminium in the body are excessive they cause the parathyroid gland to secrete more parathyroid hormone (PTH) than normal. As PTH is the substance responsible for withdrawing calcium from the bone this may lead to a whole chain of metabolic disorders. For one thing, with extra calcium circulating in the blood and soft tissue, the fragile relationship it maintains with magnesium will be disrupted. You may remember that the minerals need to be well balanced in order to work together to maintain healthy nerve cell excitability and muscle contraction. The extra calcium released by the action of aluminium on the parathyroid gland might cause the body to lose control of its muscle actions. If the victim is already suffering from Parkinson's disease, this will only help to exacerbate their muscle tremors.

In many ways the effects of aluminium on the body seem to parallel closely those of lead. It took over 2000 years for man to realize the dangers of lead. Considering that the world seems to be filling up with aluminium drinks cans and cooking utensils does this mean that we are in serious danger? No one is quite certain. The aluminium used in cans, cooking foil, saucepans and the like is fairly inert. It may be that particularly acid or alkaline foods could dislodge small amounts of the metal into your food but, at the moment at least, scientists believe that there is little threat of toxicity from these products. However, certain foods and food additives do contain appreciable amounts of aluminium that can be ingested. These include certain baking powders, some processed cheeses, white flour and antacid supplements. Finally, underarm deodorants also contain aluminium.

## Arsenic

Arsenic has had a bad press. Its use as a poison in a thousand venerable murder thrillers, not to mention in Joseph Kesselring's *Arsenic And Old Lace*, has branded it irretrievably as a toxin. In fact in small amounts, the amounts generally found in the environment, it is quite harmless. Some researchers think that in minute amounts it may even be an important nutrient, participating as a co-factor in a number of enzyme systems. Higher than normal levels of arsenic have been known to cause skin problems and even cancer, while in higher levels still, of course, it is a deadly poison. Arsenic is contained in insecticides, herbicides, pesticides, wood preservatives, alloys, paints and rat poison.

# PART FIVE

# THE VITALITY FACTOR IN ACTION

## CHAPTER 15

# Osteoporosis – Bone of Contention

Elaine is a housewife in her early fifties. She has four grown up children and lives with her estate agent husband in a green belt suburb of London. One afternoon she left her house to walk to the nearby sub-post office. It was a warm day and the perfume from her neighbour's rose and lilac bushes was heavy in the air. Walking to the corner at the end of her road she stepped off the kerb intending to cross to the small terrace of shops opposite. 'The next thing I knew I was sprawled face down in the gutter,' she recalls. 'I thought, "God! I've been knocked down." Then I remembered that I'd heard a terrific cracking sound just as I'd fallen. When I tried to move it was as if a bolt had been driven through my hip pinning me to the tarmac. Then it started to hurt and I realized I'd broken something.' She was right. Her pelvis had fractured in three places. The sudden pressure on the joint caused by the simple act of stepping off the kerbside had caused the bone almost to crumble like plaster. She had just discovered in the worst way possible that she suffered from osteoporosis.

Every year in Britain more than 50,000 women find to their horror that they have osteoporosis. It is characterized by a thinning and increasing brittleness of the bones – both in the shaft and in the lining of hollow bones. Although these symptoms might have been present for many years, technically it is only diagnosed as osteoporosis once a victim has suffered a fracture. It is a complex degenerative disease which may start at any age but is most common in women after their menopause and men beyond the age of sixty-five. The bones to suffer the greatest degree of demineralization include the lower third of the back, the hips, wrists and jaw. Half the population over seventy suffers from it. Because of its severe destructive effects osteoporosis is ranked in the top ten most common causes of death.

Since osteoporosis is responsible for so much physical constriction, pain and debilitation, enormous efforts have been made over the past thirty years to develop effective treatments for combatting it. One of the popular medical therapies used today involves courses of hormone replacement. However, as we'll see later, experts are becoming increasingly doubtful about the long-term value of such treatments.

Another popular notion is that high doses of calcium will have a therapeutic and remedial effect on the bones. As we've seen already, the rationale behind calcium treatment is that osteoporosis is first and foremost a disease in which calcium is lost from the skeleton. Therefore, so the reasoning goes, give the bones what they need – calcium supplementation – and the problem will be solved. Unfortunately this is not a dependable therapy. As we've seen in preceding chapters bone absorption of calcium depends on many factors. These include optimal levels of a number of reacting vitamins and hormones as well as a balanced interaction between calcium and several other minerals, particularly magnesium and phosphorus. Considering that it is influenced by so many variables, expecting to rectify osteoporosis merely by raising one's calcium intake is clearly a gross oversimplification. On the other hand, by understanding the mechanisms by which each of these substances interact, then using this knowledge to our advantage, osteoporosis can be fought actively and successfully. In this chapter we'll see how. First, let's look at the causes of the disease.

## 1. Racial Differences

Osteoporosis is most common amongst the fair-skinned, lighter-boned peoples of northern Europe and north America. Hispanics and natives of the Mediterranean area are less vulnerable and at the bottom of the risk table are Africans and peoples with darker skins. This is partly due to the differences in exposure to sunlight of the different races – the more sunlight you absorb, the more vitamin D your body makes and the more calcium you absorb – and partly to the relative differences in bone density. As a rule, darker-skinned people have denser bones and are therefore better equipped to cope with mineral loss when it occurs.

## 2. Hormonal Changes

In addition to these geographical differences men are also much less likely to experience osteoporosis than women. This is because men are spared the relatively sudden and drastic hormonal changes that women must endure when they pass through the menopause. The decline in oestrogen production that results from the menopause, and the knock-on effect on other hormonal secretions which are responsible for bone storage is the single most important cause of osteoporosis. For example, oestrogen acts as an inhibitory hormone on the parathyroid gland. Without adequate oestrogen this gland is free to secrete parathyroid hormone (PTH) in larger amounts. As we saw in Chapter 4, PTH determines the rate at which calcium is reabsorbed from the bone back into the blood and soft tissues. The more PTH, the faster the rate of reabsorption and consequent bone loss. Osteoporosis usually begins to show between ten and twenty years after the menopause or, if menopause has been induced surgically with the removal of the ovaries, within as little as four years.

## 3. Dangerous Habits

Although this drop in oestrogen is the most common cause of osteoporosis there are many other contributory factors which often work together to increase the chances of acute bone loss occurring. Women smokers, for example, develop osteoporosis on average five years earlier in their lives than non-smokers, and the rate of their bone loss once it starts is a staggering (literally) 50 per cent greater. While everyone accepts that smoking causes heart disease and cancer few people realize that the damage it causes is so widespread that no part of the body's metabolism is safe. For instance, vitamin C is a crucial element in building the protein matrices of collagen into which the minerals calcium and phosphate are slotted; yet it is estimated that a single cigarette will destroy up to 45 mgs of vitamin C. So a relatively modest 20 cigarettes a day uses up more of your body's vitamin C than the government recommends you eat. And if a woman drinks heavily as well as smokes the nutritional dice become even more heavily loaded against her – bone loss in a heavy drinker under forty-five years of age is comparable with that of a non-drinking osteoporosis victim in her late sixties.

Anorexics often suffer osteoporosis. Since bone loss can be triggered by a deficiency of any single nutrient essential for bone storage (such as vitamin C) think how much greater the chances of developing the disease are when the body is systematically starved of not one but every nutrient. And, as anorexia may also interfere with menstruation, oestrogen production will decline as well, providing osteoporosis with another potential foothold in the body.

## 4. Dietary Factors

At the opposite end of the spectrum to anorexia, high protein diets can also hinder mineral absorption and lead to bone loss. Eskimos, who exist almost exclusively on the meat of fish and seals, suffer one of the highest incidences of osteoporosis in the world. Vegetarians who obtain their protein from cheese and eggs, on the other hand, have much stronger, more resilient bones.

Poorly chosen, inadequately nutritious food is popular among young people. We saw at length in Chapter 3 how even seemingly well balanced diets can lead to deficiencies. Since the diets of many teenagers and young adults consist largely of fast food, carbonated drinks and sweets, their diets are anything but well balanced and the dangers are consequently that much greater. Despite occurring mainly in the elderly, osteoporosis is no respecter of youth and even if the symptoms don't become apparent at the time, these unbalanced foods can light the metabolic equivalent of a slow burning fuse. It may take many years but at some point the imbalances they have triggered could cause osteoporosis.

## 5. Digestion

Low stomach acid is another important contributing cause of osteoporosis. Calcium can only be absorbed into the body from an upper section of the small intestine near the stomach and in an acid environment. As we age our levels of stomach acid decline rapidly. In women this can become very serious after the menopause for an inability to absorb calcium might easily combine with oestrogen loss to aggravate the drop in calcium levels of the bone. The decline in stomach acid secretions is not confined to the elderly, though. Many people use antacid tablets regularly as a sort of final course to their meals and this is disastrous for their digestion. Inevitably, smoking also depletes the body of stomach acid.

## 6. Lack of Exercise

Another contributing factor to bone loss which is symptomatic of ageing is the way that many people's lifestyles become more sedentary. Yet physical activity is as important in the elderly as it is at any time of life, for a lack of exercise will also lead to bone loss. As the American nutritionist Grace Harstad observes: 'Bone growth requires the expenditure of effort against the resistance of gravity.' This expenditure of effort is vital in ensuring that the bone matrices receive a continuing supply of food and oxygen. For unlike static minerals, the collagen matrices which support them are dynamic structures of living protein in a state of constant flux. To perform their job, therefore, they must be fed. And like every protein in the body they receive what they need from the blood. Unlike most other parts of the body, though, the flow of blood through the bone is determined only in part by the pumping action of the heart. The bones themselves complete the process. When they are moved by the muscles the blood is forced through the tiny vessels in the bone much as water is moved by an old, hand-operated pump. At least half an hour's exercise a day, even if it is only a brisk walk, is essential for ensuring that the blood flows efficiently through the bones.

Without such exercise the blood pressure will build up inside the bone matrices and this will trigger the formation of cells called osteoclasts whose job is to reduce the pressure. They do this by actually dissolving the matrix, eating their way through the bone almost like woodworm through a timbered beam, so allowing the blood to escape.

### 7. Stress

Stress also has a major bearing on the health of your bones. The hormonal changes that are triggered during stress cause the marrow inside the bones to produce blood platelets that are more sticky than usual and tend to clump together. These clumps are called microthrombi and as they coalesce they form a thick sludge in the small blood vessels of the bone. Then, with less space available for the blood to flow through, pressure builds up in the matrix leading, once again, to the formation of osteoclasts and the enforced breakdown of the bone. This stress-related breakdown is rare in younger bodies, which more easily regulate and resist the production of the osteoporosis-inducing hormones, but becomes more of a risk as we age.

Another harmful substance released during stress is called the corticosteroid hormone and it prevents the bone from remodelling itself. Artificial variants of corticosteroids – such as cortisone – are sometimes prescribed for autoimmune diseases in the elderly such as rheumatism. However, when present with other factors common in old age like lack of exercise, microthrombi, stress and low stomach acid, they may increase the likelihood of osteoporosis-related fractures by up to nine times.

Other contributing causes include a deficiency of the calcium-absorbing vitamin D in your diet, perhaps as a result of too little sunlight, or sustained use of antibiotics or diuretics.

## The Effects of Osteoporosis

What happens when you develop osteoporosis? How will you know that you have it? An early symptom is periodontal disease, since the jaw is the first bone in the body to lose minerals. The gums might become inflamed and begin to bleed while at the same time receding away from the teeth, causing them to loosen in their sockets.

Then, as the collagen matrices degrade and the calcium leaches out of the bones, a victim might experience a dull pain throughout the body. However, since the pain is very similar to the sort of aching one experiences before the onset of flu, it might easily be misdiagnosed as a viral complaint. In fact since at least 30 per cent of the skeleton's calcium must be lost before osteoporosis shows up on an x-ray it is difficult to pinpoint the disease in its early stages. Blood tests are fruitless as people have been known to suffer from a 50 per cent loss of calcium from the bones while their blood calcium levels have appeared perfectly normal. As we saw with Elaine at the start of the chapter the osteoporosis might develop completely unrecognized until it caused a serious fracture. For with the bones becoming fragile, brittle and porous, it might only require a relatively innocuous jarring of a joint to lead to breakage. Another common symptom is a loss of height and, in extreme but by no means rare cases, the so-called dowager's hump resulting from the outright collapse of one of the vertebrae. So what can be done for the victims?

## The Pros and Cons of Oestrogen

Perhaps the most popular form of osteoporosis treatment is hormone replacement therapy (HRT), in which women who have passed beyond the menopause and whose subsequent decline in oestrogen secretion has led to bone loss, are administered high replacement doses of oestrogen. Few people doubt the ability of HRT to substantially slow down bone loss. Oestrogen is, after all, one of those substances which the body uses for keeping secretions of PTH – the calcium reabsorption hormone – at a manageable level. Therefore, by inhibiting PTH release, this additional oestrogen acts to help keep the calcium where it belongs: in the bones.

But is admitting that HRT slows down bone loss the same as saying that it benefits osteoporosis sufferers? Apparently not, according to Dr Ellen Grant. In her book, *The Bitter Pill*, Dr Grant says that although tests show that women taking oestrogen after the menopause do not lose bone so quickly, little mention is made about the huge drop-out rates of women on the therapy and why most of them stop taking the hormone within two or three years.

To explain the disparity between the claims of HRT supporters and the facts implicit in such a high drop-out rate, Dr Grant cites two contrasting American studies involving oestrogen replacement. One study, conducted at Harvard University, produced figures to support the claim that oestrogen usage after the menopause worked to reduce the rate of heart disease. Yet, in contradiction, the other study, conducted by the Framingham Heart Study group, concluded that oestrogen given to post-menopausal women raised their chances of heart disease by 50 per cent and fully doubled their chances of suffering a stroke. On closer examination the methods used to conduct these two studies differed greatly. While the Framingham group selected women from a comprehensively wide range of ages and health, Harvard was more selective in who it used and sometimes excluded women from any further testing once it was discovered they had coronary disease or cancer.

Since it has been found that HRT can lead to symptoms as varied as dizziness, thrombosis, cancer of the womb, varicose veins, anxiety, depression and schizophrenia is it any wonder that very few women use it for longer than three years? In fact, ironically, HRT may even cause osteoporosis. This is partly due to the fact that doctors are now combining oestrogen with progesterone – the other hormone found in the Pill – to lessen the risk of cancer of the womb. Yet, although the chances of cancer may be reduced by this combination, when given as HRT these two hormones lead to the formation of microthrombi in the bone. As we've seen, these sticky clumps of blood platelets will quickly lead to the breakdown of bone – and a shortcut to osteoporosis.

## The Calcium Craze

The other popular osteoporosis treatment today is, of course, calcium supplementation. We saw in Chapter 4 how the craze for calcium has swept America like a bushfire. Calcium is now catching on in Britain. In fact, despite calcium's unquestioned popularity, the notion of calcium supplementation as a cure for osteoporosis is nowhere near the cut and dried issue it appears. To begin with, a good number of the calcium supplements on the market may have a positively detrimental effect on your health.

For instance, TUMS, a widely used antacid supplement, has been promoted by various women's organizations across America as the solution for osteoporosis. Ye this supplement actively neturalizes the body's stomach acid, acid which is vital in helping the lining of the small intestine to absorb the calcium. Since the largest proportion of those taking supplements are the elderly, that group with the lowest levels of stomach acid to begin with, taking TUMS regularly could prove very damaging. In addition, the calcium in TUMS comes in a salt form called calcium carbonate. This is the same substance that forms as scale on kettle elements in hard water areas. Although the body is able to absorb small amounts of it, the comparatively large quantities taken in supplemental form – particularly in a low acid environment – merely pass straight through the alimentary canal. Bone meal is another badly-absorbed calcium supplement, mainly because of its poor solubility. It has a low calcium potency and is therefore hardly worth taking in the first place. Additionally, some users of bone meal have experienced blood toxicity as the animals from which the bone was obtained have had a high lead content.

Even when you do find a calcium supplement which is worth its salt such as calcium lactate or calcium gluconate (see Chapter 20 for a full list of supplements and their potency) the next question to ask is: Will it really relieve my osteoporosis? The answer is a qualified no, the reason being that, despite all the fuss and furore over calcium, osteoporosis is primarily not a problem of calcium intake. Many victims of the disease ingest perfectly healthy leavels of calcium yet still suffer the inexorable agony of bone loss. In other words, we have to look beyond calcium for relief. You may remember in Chapter 4 how we examined the relationship between the intake of calcium and its degree of absorption into the bone. We found that the amount of calcium eaten had very little bearing on the density of your bones. What matters are the indirect nutritional factors such as the levels of magnesium, vitamin D and phosphorus.

Magnesium, in particular, is also responsible for stimulating the calcium storage hormone, calcitonin. But since calcium antagonizes magnesium, raising your calcium levels through supplementation while ignoring magnesium may act directly to reduce the levels of calcitonin. And, at the same time, this drop in magnesium encourages an increase in the circulating levels of PTH – the bone reabsorption hormone. Therefore, if you decide to take calcium as a supplement, at the very least you should take the equivalent proportion of supplemental magnesium. Some nutritionists recommend a ratio of one to one. The more enlightened supplement manufacturers are now producing a combined calcium/magnesium supplement (see Chapter 20) and this appears by far the best way of obtaining additional calcium. It goes a long way to ensuring that the calcium is stored in your bones where you need it, rather than swilling dangerously around in the soft tissue.

Vitamin D is another substance which must be taken into account. It is the chemical which ensures that calcium is absorbed through the wall of the small intestine and if you increase your calcium intake you have to do likewise with vitamin D. However, nutritionally, vitamin D is a double-edged sword and if taken in excess may do permanent damage. For one thing it is a natural antagonist of magnesium and you must be careful about how much you take. The only way to determine how much you might need is through a blood test.

Another antagonist is phosphorus, depressing not only magnesium levels but, when present in excess, causing the bone to get rid of its calcium. Since phosphorus is normally present in our diets in high amounts there seems to be no reasonable call for phosphorus supplementation. On the contrary, we recommend that you cut down on foods which are high in phosphorus (see Chapter 6 for a list of these foods).

In summary: osteoporosis is caused by many different factors, all of which must be taken into account. Simply using one of the popular treatments to obtain relief is far from satisfactory. For it only deals with one small aspect of the problem – the tip of the iceberg, if you like – while, unseen, the real problem penetrates deep to the very heart of the body's intricate metabolic pathways. Surely it is better to think of treatments that look to rectify body-wide problems. Let's look at a list of things you can do to get right to the heart of the matter. This list forms a good preventative programme as well as helping to keep symptoms at bay if you already suffer from osteoporosis.

## 1. Assess Your Mineral Profile

To determine how balanced your intake of calcium, magnesium and phosphorus is, refer to the lists of foods which contain those minerals. You'll find them in Chapter 6. If, for example, you drink large quantities of carbonated drinks and habitually eat a lot of red meat, your phosphorus level could well be too high in relation to the other minerals. You might, for example, feel the need to increase your magnesium sources – either through a careful choice of foods or by supplementation – whilst decreasing those of phosphorus. By carefully regulating your mineral intake you can play an active, hands-on role in helping these mineral levels to stay where they belong.

As we've seen, there are many more minerals involved in bone metabolism than just three. Zinc, for example, is also important for bone growth as it is used in the formation of the bone collagen matrix. Manganese, too, helps to maintain healthy bones as well as guarding against malformation. Therefore, a test to establish the overall ratio of these minerals is very important. For example, imagine your test reveals an excess of copper. Since copper antagonizes zinc, it would be reasonable to assume that a certain amount of zinc, which is necessary for collagen formation, was being lost from the body. Therefore, even if your calcium-magnesium-phosphorus ratio were perfect, lack of zinc would hinder healthy bone formation. Having found this out, it would be a comparatively simple thing to cut down on copper-rich foods and raise your zinc levels through supplementation. The same goes for any depleted mineral. (For details of the different mineral tests available and the different supplements see Chapters 19 and 20 respectively).

## 2. Assessing Your Diet as a Whole

It is also important to take other groups of food into account. A low-fibre diet, for example, will hinder mineral absorption. So will eating too much protein. For when the gut contains more protein than it can digest, a layer of mucus forms on the digestive tract walls. This has two effects: firstly, it provides a home for unfriendly and potentially dangerous bacteria and secondly it acts as a barrier, preventing the minerals from being absorbed. Always try to ensure that your diet is rich in high-fibre foods. If you eat a lot of protein why not cut down a little, perhaps by eating one less meat meal a week?

## 3. Improving your digestion

There is a popular saying that you are what you eat. More accurately, though admittedly more clumsily, you are what you digest of what you eat. Your digestive ability is a crucial factor in evaluating how well you are absorbing all the nutrients essential for healthy bones. As people approach middle age their ability to manufacture stomach acid frequently declines and sometimes disappears altogether. Yet stomach acid is critically important in helping the body to absorb its food, particularly minerals such as calcium and magnesium which depend on an acid environment. Even if you raise your mineral intake by regulating your diet or through supplementation, without adequate acid the minerals will simply pass through the gut unabsorbed. One study which examined how successfully two of the most popular forms of calcium supplementation – dolomite and bone meal – were absorbed showed that in those people whose stomach acid levels had declined appreciably no extra calcium was obtained at all. And stomach acid is not only important for digestion in its own right, it also stimulates the pancreas into secreting enzymes for completing digestion further down the gut.

If a mineral analysis test (see pages 165–9 for details) shows that many of your body's minerals are low even though you are following a balanced diet then it is a fair guess that your digestion is functioning poorly. There are three useful tests for evaluating your digestive ability. The first is a gastrogram which indicates the stomach's ability to generate stomach acid. The second is a stool analysis. This reveals your overall ability to digest food, its fibre content, and the levels of friendly and unfriendly bacteria. The third is swallowing a capsule of vegetable dye. The resulting colour of your urine gives an indication of how well the capsule has been dissolved.

You might wonder after reading this just what your digestion has to do with osteoporosis. If so then you've been influenced by the attitudes of conventional medicine which condition us to think of the different parts and functions of the body as independent operations in their own right. In fact they are interdependent parts of a whole. If one part suffers, the whole body suffers. And conversely, for total health you need to treat the whole body.

## 4. Other nutritional supplementation

This metabolic overview also extends to nutrients in the body other than minerals. Take protein, for instance. You may remember that when we looked at calcium in Chapter 4 we met a protein-like substance called calmodulin. This molecule works with calcium by helping it to adapt to a variety of uses related to nerve and cell function, blood clotting and bone mineralization. Calmodulin, therefore, is one of the most important factors in preventing a buildup of calcium where it is not needed. Protein is also used by the bones to manufacture the collagen matrices into which calcium and phosphorus are built. And finally, the body builds its digestive enzymes from protein, enzymes which the gut must have in order to break down and digest the minerals and other nutrients from its food.

An excellent way of ensuring that your body receives all the protein it needs is by taking a free-form amino acid supplement. Free-form amino acids are the tiny constituent molecules of every protein in your body. There are approximately twenty amino acids and you can obtain them as a complete blend in one supplement. As the basic constituents of protein they are not thought of as a medicine but as a food. However, unlike protein, which is obtained from sources such as meat, they supply your body with the nutrition it needs without hindering the digestion and absorption of minerals. We're not suggesting that you substitute free-form aminos for all your protein, but if you decide to cut down your protein intake then amino acids are a high-powered nutritional insurance against any protein depletion. (See Chapter 20 for a list of amino acid suppliers.)

As well as protein, certain vitamins are also most important for generating strong bones. We've already looked at vitamin D. Another useful vitamin is C. This is a vital component in collagen formation and you would be well advised to take as much as a gramme of vitamin C in supplemental form with each meal. This is never more important than when you smoke.

For many people, osteoporosis seems to strike with a brutal inevitability. However, by following these guidelines you can drastically raise your resistance to this awful disease. No one is pretending that they are easy and convenient to follow, far from it. But with patience and application – regulating your mineral intake, ensuring that your digestion is healthy and feeding your metabolic pathways with all the nutrients they need – you can protect yourself against osteoporosis like never before.

# CHAPTER 16

# Mid-Life and Beyond

Whilst osteoporosis has occasionally been known to afflict the young many years before their bodies undergo the mid-life hormonal changes, it is a disease that generally occurs sometime after the menopause has taken place. And it is particularly rife among the elderly, that group of people who are most vulnerable to nutrition-related disorders. Although osteoporosis is the most highly publicized of such disorders, it is only one of many that occur as the body ages. In this chapter we'll look at some of the others and see how mineral supplementation may be able to help.

When a person ages, their body's hormonal activity decreases as a natural consequence. This means that cellular activity, in the form of its millions of metabolic pathways, slows down in the same way that a car changes into progressively lower gears. An ageing body might, in effect, be content to chug along in second gear when, in its youth, it might easily have coasted along in fourth. As the metabolic rate slows, certain functions cease altogether. Growth, for example, is halted while the neverending processes of maintenance and regeneration of cells, processes that are vital to the health of the body, are reduced to a minimum. At the same time the degenerative processes of oxidation increase and start to overtake this declining regenerative activity. This is what causes the body to age. It allows the bones to soften, the skin to wrinkle and the hair to coarsen; it leaves the body less resistant to infection and robs it of its strength and energy.

Ageing is inevitable but the speed with which it affects the body is not. With a carefully chosen diet, a diet that wherever possible avoids processed foods in favour of much more nutritious, unprocessed, freshly prepared foods, the effects of age can be staved off for many years and the body's youth and vigour maintained.

## Ageing Versus Nutrition

However, in ensuring that the body receives all the vitamins, minerals and proteins needed to sustain your youthful vitality you cannot help but run headlong into a paradox. On the one side the body's need for nutrients increases as it ages; yet on the other, with its metabolic rate slowing, its need for calories diminishes. Nutritionists estimate that a 70-year-old woman requires only 50 per cent of the calories needed by her 20-year-old granddaughter. Yet, if the grandmother is to resist successfully the ravages of ageing, her need for nutrients equals, and may even exceed, her granddaughter's. If the 70-year-old were to consume the same amount of food as the 20-year-old, the sluggish rate at which her body would metabolize the food and burn the energy it contains would lead to a buildup of cholesterol in the blood vessels and tissue. This could cause heart disease, circulatory disorders and obesity, all of which will encourage the ageing process to accelerate.

Here we have the most compelling argument possible for using nutritional supplementation. For, while it might conceivably be possible to obtain all the nutrition you need for your diet when you are young, it is almost impossible to do the same once your body enters into mid-life with its declining calorie needs. Supplements, on the other hand, provide the body with optimal amounts of vital nutrients without a concomitant increase in calorie intake. For this reason minerals make particularly effective anti-ageing fighters. Let's see which are the best.

## 1. Iodine

The first priority when using mineral supplementation to prolong your body's youthful vitality is to try and minimize the decline in hormonal activity. We saw in the previous chapter how a carefully balanced combination of minerals, including calcium and magnesium, enhances and prolongs the role played by the hormone oestrogen in strengthening the bone. Iodine can help to do the same with the thyroid gland by stimulating thyroxin secretion. As you know, by secreting thyroxin, the thyroid gland determines the rate at which our bodies burn and release energy, as well as the degree of cell growth and reproduction.

Iodine is a key component of both thyroxin and the thyroid gland itself. Severe deficiency of this mineral causes goitre, lethargy, poor healing, a low resistance to disease and a lack of mental focus. In the same way, as we age and less thyroxin is secreted, our muscle tone slackens and energy levels decrease, while a high level of concentration becomes more difficult to attain. In addition, fat starts to build up beneath the skin and in the arteries. The living functions of the body effectively start to wind down. However, by stimulating the production of additional thyroxin, iodine supplementation can help to slow down this process. Elderly patients who have been put on a long-term programme of iodine supplementation report renewed energy and enthusiasm for life coupled with a substantial loss of excess fat. In addition, researchers find that it increases mental alertness and in some cases even leads to more pliant skin.

Of course, it's not the iodine alone that does all this. We've stressed time and again throughout the book the importance firstly of minerals as a biochemical family, and secondly as part of the body's overall nutritional needs, needs that include vitamins, proteins and fatty acids. Iodine is not a panacea. Even though it may encourage the body's thyroxin levels to rise, all the nutrients necessary for healthy metabolism need to be present to take advantage of the situation. This means providing the body with supplements of each important mineral in their most easily assimilable form. Chapter 20 lists the recommended forms of minerals available while on pages 172–4 you'll find a complete formulation that you may like to follow in order to give your body optimal amounts of the most easily assimilated minerals.

## 2. Zinc

Among the commonest of age-related disorders in men are the problems involving the prostate gland. It's not unusual for middle-aged and elderly men to suffer either from an atrophied or a swollen prostate (this is also known as prostitis). Either state can disrupt bladder function, lead to impotence, cause severe, debilitating pain and in extreme cases even lead to cancer. The prostate gland, which is situated just below the bladder, secretes seminal fluid. Often the amount of zinc lost in an ejaculation exceeds a man's daily intake. Therefore, if a man is sexually active, the cumulative loss of zinc substantially increases his risk of developing prostate disease, especially if his diet is heavily processed and refined.

Some nutritionists speculate that there is a connection between loss of zinc from the prostate and loss of iodine from the thyroid gland. In the case of the thyroid it is an established medical fact that iodine deficiency leads to the swelling we know as goitre. Could it be that in the same way a loss of zinc over many years leads to the swelling of prostitis? No one is willing to say for certain, at least not yet, but there is mounting evidence in the form of case histories to back up this supposition. One such case involved Andy, an organic farmer in his late fifties who, for the previous twenty years had been a vegan, living mainly from his own organically grown produce. Andy was first troubled by prostate trouble when he experienced difficulty urinating, coupled with minor but irritating bladder incontinence. Occasionally, he'd also experience a short stabbing pain in the genital area. Gradually the problem grew worse, the pain becoming more intense and lasting for longer periods while he occasionally lost control of his bladder altogether. During this time he also became impotent. His doctor diagnosed acute prostitis and recommended surgery as the only sure means of relief.

As an organic farmer, Andy had long been involved with, and interested in, alternative forms of health care. He decided that rather than simply accept his doctor's opionion he would have his body's nutritional profile analysed. A hair analysis showed low mineral levels across the board but his zinc levels were discovered to be particularly low. A negative result from the Bryce-Smith test, which determines the body's zinc content using the sense of taste (see page 169 for details), confirmed that he was suffering from drastically low zinc levels. Andy attributed this to his limited diet and an over-dependence on one sort of soil. If the soil on his farm was, as he suspected, depleted of zinc, then the fact that most of his diet was obtained from food grown in this soil would mean that the depletion was passed on to him. Andy was put on a course of 50 mg of zinc citrate a day together with vitamin B6 to help metabolize the zinc and the supplemental back-up of the entire mineral formulation (see pages 172–4).

Within two months Andy's symptoms had all but disappeared. In addition he and his wife were understandably delighted with the resulting rise in his libido. 'Everyone I'd spoken to, including my doctor, had told me that my problems were an inevitable product of ageing,' Andy said. 'I'd come to believe myself that it was quite common for a man of my age to develop prostate trouble, not to mention lose interest in sex, and not be able to do anything about it. I realize now just how complacent and misleading this view is.'

While zinc is good for men to help counteract the effects of prostate trouble as well as enhance sexual potency, both sexes need zinc to combat the growing threat to the body of environmental pollution. Most forms of smoke carry with them dangerous heavy metals, free radical agents which antagonize the body's essential minerals, destroy vitamins and break down numerous enzyme systems. Perhaps the smoke to which we are all most commonly exposed is that of tobacco, with its high cadmium content. As we saw in chapters 8 and 13, cadmium antagonizes zinc and in doing so ravages the body's soft tissue. Not surprisingly, smoking is today one of the foremost clues of premature ageing and of illnesses such as bronchitis, emphysema and lung cancer – all of which most commonly afflict victims in later life. Nutritionists have found that zinc supplementation, by preventing the absorption of free radicals, is highly effective at reducing the risk of contracting these diseases.

## 3. Selenium

Like zinc, selenium also assists the body by protecting vulnerable tissue from free radical damage. You may remember from chapter 10 that selenium is an essential component of glutathione peroxidase (GTP), an enzyme that functions as one of the body's most important free radical defences. Without adequate selenium your body would be unable to manufacture GTP in sufficient quantities to protect itself from the many varieties of environmental pollution that contribute to the ageing process.

Selenium's enormous preventative effect on cancer, one of the greatest scourges of the elderly, has been demonstrated time and again. Studies show that populations living in areas, and following diets, high in selenium have a significantly lower incidence rate of cancer. It is particularly effective in enhancing skin vitality and researchers also believe that it makes a huge contribution to the ability of your immune system to resist disease and infection.

Matthew, a retired engineer, was recently diagnosed as suffering from cancer of the saliva gland and his doctor had no alternative but to have the organ removed. What the doctor was unable to do, that Matthew found frustrating, was suggest a possible cause of the cancer or guarantee that it wouldn't spread to other parts of the body. Since Matthew had made a career out of problem-solving he determined to unearth the roots of his illness. In the course of his research he came across hair analysis and decided to have such a test performed on himself. The results were dramatic, showing mercury levels far beyond anything the laboratory conducting the test had ever encountered. This was almost certainly the cause of Matthew's cancer, especially when he traced the source to a tonic that he had drunk religiously for thirty years. A nutritionist recommended he take selenium in two forms, sodium selenate and selenium 1-methionine (see page 174) as well as vitamin C to aid in precipitating the mercury out of his body. Matthew had taken the tonic for so long that it was simply impossible to guarantee that he wouldn't in future be harmed by the cumulative effects of all that mercury. However, by following a strictly regimented diet together with the essential nutritional support of selenium, Matthew has taken the best possible precaution in his efforts to prevent the cancer from spreading.

Since it is such an integral part of the body's defences against environmental toxicity, selenium may also work in the body as an allergy-fighter. In her book *Ageless Ageing* the health writer Leslie Kenton highlights the report of a group of chemical ecologists who tested selenium on a group of men and women all of whom had been diagnosed as suffering from the effects of environmentally related allergies. In complex trials the researchers discovered that selenium supplementation alone was able to clear up the symptoms in 60 per cent of their patients.

Since many scientists see allergies as one of the major causes of age-related bone disorders such as rheumatism and arthritis, selenium could prove to be one of the most effective of all anti-ageing supplements. What is more, it will protect the bones from these diseases in two quite distinct ways, firstly be reducing the effects of allergy, and secondly by preventing the oxidation and consequent rancidity, of essential fatty acids by pollution-generated free radicals. Essential fatty acids are important for helping to lubricate and cushion the cells in the ligaments and joints. When these fatty acids become rancid – going off in the same way that butter or milk will go off – the result will be the easily recognized and much dreaded symptoms of rheumatism: the gnawing, grinding, immobilizing pain. By blocking the action of the free radicals, and thus preventing rancidity, selenium will help you to avoid this. Don't forget it is best taken with its synergist vitamin E.

## Assiduous Acid

One special aspect of ageing that must be taken into account when dealing with nutrition is the decline in the body's production of stomach acid as it grows older. Stomach acid is probably the single most important substance in the whole digestive process. It destroys any bacteria that we inadvertently swallow with our food, keeps the gut's indigenous population of bacteria in check and stimulates the pancreas into secreting digestive enzymes in the intestine. Crucially, nearly all the minerals we eat can only be absorbed through the gut wall in an acid environment. The less stomach acid the body has available, the fewer minerals it will absorb. In order to help the body realize its full potential in its fight against ageing it is absolutely crucial that it absorbs all the minerals it can. This means ensuring that the body has sufficient stomach acid to do the job. Yet, by the age of sixty-five, almost a third of the population have no stomach acid left at all. Luckily health shops are now stocking supplements which contain the hydrochloric acid necessary for facilitating digestion. If your local health food shop doesn't stock these supplements, see page 174 for the addresses of suppliers that do.

CHAPTER 17

# Circulatory Problems

It is hardly surprising that we refer to main roads in Britain as arterial highways. For blood vessels are to your body what the road and rail networks are to the country. They are the most widely used means of giving nutrients to the cells, quickly and with a minimum of wasted energy. Oxygen is collected from the lungs by the red corpuscles and dispersed throughout the body in the arteries. Then, in turn, it is the veins' job to return the used oxygen in the form of carbon dioxide back to the lungs. At the same time, the nutrients obtained from food filters through to the blood from the gut and are carried to wherever they are needed. And, just as our roads have a mobile police force to collar and penalize offenders, so the blood has its own defences in the form of white blood cells, the shock troops of the body's immune system.

Our circulatory system can be compared to two sinuous rivers, winding their way in opposite directions, often parallel but never touching, through a dense landscape. One river contains blood that has been saturated with oxygen from the lungs. And it seems to be flowing backwards. From the wide, shallow delta of the membranous lung tissue it becomes a strong, surging current before separating into smaller and smaller tributaries. These are the arteries and in turn they divide into minute filaments called capillaries. By the time this division reaches its limit these arterial vessels are little more in diameter than the width of a molecule and they feed their oxygen straight into the cell. In turn, other minute capillaries receive carbon dioxide as a waste product of the energy burning process before starting their long trek back to the lungs – where they deposit the waste – this time as tributaries of the second river system, the veins.

In summary, the health of your blood vessels – their pliancy, ability to smoothly contract and relax, and their freedom from constriction and blockage – are as important to your health as the life blood which they carry. Consequently, when anything happens to damage the vessels, or harm the oxygen and nutrient-carrying blood, the results in terms of ill-health can be widespread and, in many cases, mortally dangerous. Heart disease, for example, is Britain's largest single killer, while strokes and haemorrhages resulting from blocked or constricted vessels also create their share of debilitation and death. Anaemia, too, is a common blood-related illness.

One of the most serious circulatory problems – particularly, but by no means exclusively, in older patients – is the buildup of fatty plaques in the blood vessels. Plaque is debris, composed primarily of cholesterol and certain minerals, that results from inadequate food metabolism and an unbalanced diet. Take, for example, the habit of eating too much of the wrong kinds of fat, such as the saturated fatty acids in red meat. Since the body can only make limited use of this kind of fat it often accumulates in large amounts in the blood. The body does have enzymes to cope with this situation, but too often it is simply unable to break down such large quantities.

A second contributing factor is the increase in body levels of certain minerals which, once absorbed, have nowhere to go and nothing to do. Calcium is, of course, the prime example since so many people are unwisely increasing their calcium intake without considering the effects this may have on the body. Therefore, by not taking into account the importance of synergists, such as magnesium, which ensure that this extra calcium will be stored where it is needed, it will circulate in the blood like a lonely child traipsing the streets late at night. Until it falls in with bad company. The influence that turns it to delinquency in this case is the contact with those fats.

The result of this contact is a molecule called calcium phospholipid. It is inert, sticky, sludgelike and – crucially – insoluble. It will adhere on the blood vessel walls and attract more molecules of the same substance as they pass, creating a lump, or plaque, that grows progressively larger.

Whilst this is taking place the day-by-day reactions of the body continue apace. Blood is pulsed around the body constantly, feeding the cells and removing waste products for safe disposal by the kidneys. Now, though, it must contend with the plaques. As they grow they begin to constrict the space in the vessel available for the passage of blood, forcing the heart to pump more quickly and vigorously simply to push the blood around at the same rate as before. This rate is vital for ensuring that the cells' oxygen supply is renewed quickly and regularly, yet maintaining the rate in the face of the obstacles mounted by the plaques means submitting to a rise in blood pressure. The stresses which this puts on the heart may at first lead to dizziness and breathlessness, later to the cramping chest pains of angina. Finally, it may cause a heart attack as the poor overworked heart simply gives up the ghost, in the same way that your leg muscles might develop cramp and give way beneath you after a bout of overstrenuous activity.

The blood vessels themselves also suffer. The initial buildup of plaques is known as atherosclerosis and is a dangerous enough condition in its own right. In time, thought, it also leads to arteriosclerosis, a state where the vessel walls themselves become damaged. Picture a slow-moving river. It meanders its way across the countryside, snaking this way and that with only slow and minimal bank erosion. Now picture a fast-moving torrent, tearing chunks of the bank away with it, often even overflowing the banks itself. The difference between these two rivers and their banks is the difference between the blood, and blood vessels, of someone with clear arteries and someone with plaque-induced atherosclerosis. The more chronic the atherosclerosis, the higher the blood pressure and the greater the damage inflicted on the vessel walls. In time this damage causes the walls to harden and reduces their pliancy. This is known as arteriosclerosis. How can minerals help?

## 1. Sodium Ascorbate

A number of medicines exist which remove plaques from the vessel walls. Don't forget, though, that these plaques are insoluble and once they lose their anchorages they simply drift for a while before settling elsewhere. The problem, therefore, doesn't so much disappear as relocate itself. However, an English scientist, Sherry Lewin, has found one substance that not only removes plaque from blood vessel walls but also affects it in such a way that it can be dissolved and safely disposed. This substance is vitamin C. Crucially, it is one of the three available mineral forms of the vitamin that achieves this remarkable feat – sodium ascorbate. When sodium ascorbate circulates in the bloodstream it combines with calcium phospholipid to produce sodium phospholipid and calcium ascorbate, both of which are soluble.

Humans are one of the few species unable to manufacture vitamin C in their bodies and this is a contributing factor to their vulnerability to high blood pressure, atherosclerosis and related problems (other factors, of course, include stress and poor diet). Another such animal is the lowly guinea pig. By withholding sodium ascorbate from the diets of a group of guinea pigs a research scientist, Emil Getner, recently found that their arteries quickly began to clog and harden. When he gave the animals additional amounts of sodium ascorbate, however, their symptoms faded.

It is likely that the dredging and dissolving effect of sodium ascorbate would be accelerated by supplemental magnesium. This mineral is, of course, calcium's uneasy metabolic partner. The more magnesium the body ingests, the more calcium the bones will absorb, so preventing a buildup of plaque in the blood vessels.

## 2. Magnesium and calcium

In fact, the influence of magnesium extends far beyond its involvement in the restriction of plaque. You may remember from Chapter 5 that we saw how magnesium plays a crucial role in nerve excitability, particularly in terms of muscle contraction and relaxation. Ionic magnesium acts as a sort of transformer, reducing and regulating the strength of a message as it passes from the nerves to the muscles. This protects the body from oversusceptibility to stimuli, and ensures that the muscles don't overrespond when they receive the stimuli. If the body is magnesium-deficient, however, the reverse happens. As far as the circulatory system is concerned this may mean an increased heart rate, higher blood pressure and an irregular beat. And it may lead in time to the problems of atherosclerosis and arteriosclerosis that we've already examined.

Of course, magnesium is only one of two minerals that work together as nerve regulators. The other is calcium and a deficiency or an excess (which latter under the circumstances is more likely) of this mineral will lead to to the same problems. We saw in Chapter 15 just how important a balanced intake of these two minerals is for guarding against bone disorders. Precisely the same holds true for the health, efficiency and pliancy of your blood vessels.

## 3. Chromium

This mineral, too, is proving remarkably effective at helping to improve circulation. It does so as part of the glucose tolerance factor (GTF) molecule, assisting in the metabolism of sugars and fats for release as energy. The higher the body's levels of GTF, the more efficiently it will be able to utilize the fats that might otherwise accumulate in the blood vessels as plaques. Indeed, many of the most eminent researchers in the field of nutrition, such as Richard Passwater and Carl Pfeiffer, have found that low chromium is directly associated with aortic plaques and atherosclerosis.

## 4. Iron and Copper

Since iron is a major component of haemoglobin, the oxygen-carrying molecule of the red corpuscles, a lack of iron is one of anaemia's commonest causes. Anaemia is a disorder which, even if the circulatory vessels are in perfect health, will deprive the body of its essential, energy-releasing oxygen. And, in time, the heart and the muscles of the vessel walls, themselves deprived of oxygen, will begin to suffer. The results of this oxygen shortage may include angina, breathlessness, lethargy and depression, not to mention a reduced resistance to diseases and slower growth and repair of cells. This is why iron is so important. It helps to ensure that oxygen is distributed efficiently by raising the levels of haemoglobin in the blood. Remember, though, that iron, when it is not occupied, is a free radical and that taking supplements of the mineral when they are not strictly necessary may even make the body more vulnerable to illness. Happily, since iron is concentrated in the blood, its levels can be measured with a simple blood test. If you find that your iron levels do need supplementing, you would be well advised to include a supplement of copper, too. This is because the regeneration of haemoglobin depends heavily on copper and without it you may receive all the iron you need yet still find that your cells are being given an inadequate supply of oxygen.

# CHAPTER 18

# Minerals and Muscles

Minerals are crucial for ensuring the continued health and efficiency of your muscles. Muscles play several distinct, key roles in the body. The first is to facilitate movement. Anchored to the bones, they move the skeleton like a series of powerful, interlocking levers by the process of alternately contracting and relaxing. This levering action enables us to perform every movement from simply bending a finger or lifting a box to sprinting with a long, surging stride. Secondly, the muscles are crucial for pumping blood around the body. Of course, the heart is the muscle that carries primary responsibility for circulation, but muscles in the blood vessel walls also play key roles in assisting the blood's passage. Likewise, as we saw in Chapter 15, the very act of using our muscles to resist the downward force of gravity helps pump blood into our bones, nourishing them and cleansing them of the destructive osteoclasts in the process. Therefore, without adequate exercise – that is, without using our muscles as frequently and as energetically as we should – the bones will become deprived of blood, possibly hastening the process of demineralization. We can see from this that the bones, the circulatory system and the muscles make up a single, indivisible whole. Each works in harmony with, depends upon, and is in turn depended upon by the others. We've seen in previous chapters how mineral supplementation can help the bones and the blood vessels. Now it is time to see what they can do for your muscles.

## 1. Potassium

In Chapter 7 we saw how the relationship between potassium ions inside the cell and sodium ions outside is one of the most important factors in determining the contraction and relaxation of your muscles. When muscle contraction is required – that is, whenever the body has to perform any one of its many thousands of daily mechanical tasks – potassium is forced out from the cells of the muscles involved. Consequently more sodium is brought into the cell in order to balance the electrical charge. This change in the relative concentrations of the two sets of mineral ions causes an electrical message to pass through the muscle cell and the whole muscle is made to contract. Then, when contraction is no longer required the original concentration between these two minerals is re-established and the muscle relaxes.

Remember that we are not simply talking about the movement of one limb or muscle at a time. There are over a hundred separate, articulating bones in the skeleton and at any one time a large proportion of these are moving. Therefore, while some muscles of the body are contracting, others will relax. Then some of this second group of relaxed muscles may contract while some of the first start to relax, and so on. The whole system of leverages that the muscles employ to move the bones is a constantly adapting, finely tuned mechanism, enormously sensitive to the demands placed upon it. To maintain it the body needs ample supplies of both potassium and sodium.

While there are only a few situations where the body may become deprived of sodium, such as in the case of extreme dehydration, potassium deficiency is quite common. Potassium is a dwindling part of our diets today while sodium is fifty times more prominent than it was a hundred years ago. Furthermore, this imbalance is often exacerbated by people who suffer from mild dehydration – after a strenuous game of squash, for example – habitually swallowing a supplement of sodium in salt form. They think, misguidedly that loss of body fluid automatically means a loss of sodium. As we saw in Chapter 7 this is not true. What they are doing, without realizing, is helping to disrupt further the potassium/sodium balance and increase the chances of developing the symptoms they want to avoid: cramp, muscle weakness, and so on.

Potassium is essentially the muscle relaxant and when its levels sink in relation to sodium the results will include physical lassitude, severe muscle cramping and nausea. All of these symptoms are usually diagnosed as signs of sodium loss. More often than not, nothing could be further from the truth. Our bodies are well stocked with sodium. Increasingly, however, the same cannot be said of potassium. When its levels are healthy, potassium helps to ensure good muscle tone and prevents the muscles themselves from over-responding. A mild symptom of potassium deficiency is the sort of uncontrollable, but very common, nervous tic that many people might experience as a fluttering eyelid or an inability to relax a limb enough to coordinate an implement such as a pen or a snooker cue. More seriously, it can lead to high blood pressure as the heart, deprived of potassium and with too much of the excitory sodium, is made to beat more rapidly, and harder, than is needed for circulating the blood. It can cause extreme weakness in the heavy muscles of the limbs and trunk, and it may cause a decline in muscle mass. Potassium loss, in other words, will lead to an overall loss of physical tone. Muscles will lose that elastic pliancy that characterizes a fit body, becoming instead soft and flaccid; exercise will become harder with the victim prone to frequent fits of breathlessness and dizziness as the overburdened heart struggles to cope. And since potassium is also responsible for the metabolism of sugars and fats the loss of muscle tone will be accompanied by a buildup of fat.

## 2. Magnesium

As we've seen, potassium is of paramount importance for the health and wellbeing of your muscles. However, if there has been one common theme running through this book, it is that the body's vitality is achieved not by the use of individual minerals but rather by using them in an overall, harmonious balance with the rest of the mineral family. Therefore, while potassium is important for muscle relaxation and tone inside the cells, magnesium performs a similar task outside the cell. While potassium ensures that the muscle itself doesn't over-respond to a particular nerve message by refusing to relax after contracting, magnesium helps protect the cell by reducing the strength of that message before it reaches its destination. Together these two minerals can be seen as metabolic arbiters, determining exactly how much or how little the nerves and muscles should respond. They are the body's fine tuners, regulating the excitory effects on the nerves and muscles of calcium and sodium. As with potassium, body levels of magnesium tend towards the low side. In potassium's case this is due to the unhealthy dominance of sodium. In the same way, magnesium depletion is often caused by the way we load our diets with calcium to the detriment of those minerals that should work with it. And in the same way that potassium loss causes acute muscular problems, so inadequate magnesium will lead to muscle twitching, tremors, weakness and cramping.

If you decide to take potassium to help improve the tone and strength of your muscles it would be a good idea to take magnesium as well. Certain suppliers of nutritional supplementation are now manufacturing a product that includes magnesium and potassium in a single supplement.

## 3. Zinc

While magnesium and potassium ensure that the muscles function efficiently, zinc is necessary for aiding muscle growth. The importance of zinc lies in its involvement with DNA, the molecule responsible for providing the 'blueprints' for the creation of each and every substance in the body. Naturally this process is most important for the creation of muscle protein. This is because the constant stresses, wear and tear caused by hundreds of movements a minute, mean that muscle must be regenerated and replaced frequently. Since zinc is a co-factor in the enzyme that bonds RNA to DNA, allowing replication to take place, a deficiency can interfere with the production of ribosomes. In time the creation of new muscle can be impaired. What does this mean in terms of physical wellbeing?

The effects of zinc loss on the muscles are most graphically demonstrated by the case of Tony, a young graphic designer from London. Tony's hectic lifestyle, both professionally and socially, left him with little time for eating regular, balanced meals. He freely admits that even if he had the time, his interest in food and nutrition would extend no further than slamming a packet of lasagne bought at his local supermarket into the microwave. Recently, Tony joined a health club near his office and started working out vigorously at lunchtime in the gymnasium there. 'I must have been going for a fortnight before things started to go wrong,' said Tony. 'Then I woke up one morning and my entire body felt as if it had been beaten with a baseball bat. Whenever and whatever I moved there was this awful pain. It felt deep down beneath the skin as if the bones themselves were cracking.' In considerable discomfort Tony went immediately to see his doctor who was frankly at a loss what to suggest. 'It was rather funny. The doctor actually got angry with me as he had no idea what the matter was. He came out with phrases like "growing pains" (I'm twenty-five, incidentally) and "overdoing it". He actually got quite angry with me when I told him I wasn't happy with his diagnosis.'

Over the following weekend the symptoms faded but no sooner did Tony return to the gym than the pain returned. It was especially severe in his shoulders, upper arms and trunk and so incapacitating that he almost dared not move his arms away from his sides. This time he went to see a nutritional counsellor whose practice was almost next door to Tony's office. It was here that a hair analysis revealed low zinc levels. The sudden need for freshly generated muscle that the stresses of weight lifting had imposed on his metabolism had seemingly drained Tony of what little zinc he had. Once this had disappeared his muscles were no longer able to repair themselves. They literally began to tear, particularly where the stresses were greatest, at the points where they anchored themselves to the bone. This is a common problem for runners who often suffer from a condition known as shin splints when the muscles on the front of the shins sometimes tear lose from the bones. Tony was recommended a daily dosage of 30 mg of zinc citrate together with an admonition to follow a better diet. 'I'm back weight lifting again now and there has been a terrific improvement. I don't think I'll ever be in the Schwarzenegger class but at least I'm not crippling myself any more.'

## Mineral Formulations

Below we list two formulations: one which can be used exclusively to strengthen your bones, the other which can be used as part of an overall nutritional programme for wellbeing.

In the first formulation we list several different forms of the same mineral. This is because the body uses different forms for different functions. Therefore, by including a number of the most easily absorbed varieties you can ensure the best possible bio-availability. Whenever possible try to include each of these forms in your bone-strengthening programme.

Although we recommend what we feel to be the best mineral forms for you to ingest we cannot realistically suggest how much of each you should take. The factors involved in a person's metabolic individuality –including age, sex, weight, diet, and state of health – mean that a quantity of one mineral which may be perfectly adequate for you could be too little, or too much, for somene else. This is a good argument for having a mineral test performed before putting yourself on a programme of mineral supplementation. It determines which minerals are in most need of being supplemented and gives you a good idea of how much to take. However, if for some reason such a test is impractical, you would be best advised not to exceed the dosage recommended on the product label.

### 1. Calcium and Magnesium

No matter what quantities you decide on, these two are perhaps best taken in a 1:1 ratio, preferably with a small amount of vitamin D (perhaps 50 i.u. – international units) to aid absorption:

calcium aspartate
calcium gluconate
calcium lactate
calcium orotate
magnesium aspartate
magnesium orotate
magnesium thiosulphate

### 2. Overall Programme

Include all forms of calcium and magnesium (in smaller quantities than for the bone programme alone) plus:

copper gluconate

iron as ferritin
iron as ferrous gluconate
iron as ferrous glycinate

germanium

iodine as potassium iodide

manganese gluconate
manganese glycinate

molybdenum as ammonium molybdate

potassium citrate

silicon as organic silicon

selenium as seleno-methionine

zinc citrate

# PART SIX

# THE NEXT STEP

CHAPTER 19

# Mineral Testing

Throughout this book we've attempted to explain how easily mineral deficiencies can arise. If, for example, your diet is overburdened with one group of foods to the exclusion of others, or if it contains too much processed and refined food, your body may easily become depleted of essential minerals. The same is true if you live in an area of high heavy metal pollution; if the soil and water has a poor mineral content; if you have poor digestion; if you have suffered a serious illness or undergone an operation; if you take drugs such as the contraceptive pill or diuretics; or even if you habitually take a laxative. In fact, nutritionists find that mineral imbalances usually involve a combination of these factors.

If after reading this book you think that you might yourself be the victim of a deficiency or excess what should your next step be? You can, of course, go straight out and purchase or order the minerals that you feel you are deficient in (see Chapter 20 for a list of the most effective and easily assimilable forms). Alternatively you might first want to confirm your suspicions by undergoing a mineral test. There are a number of different tests available. The most commonly performed is blood analysis. Others involve examining your hair, urine or saliva. Each test has its good points in the way it shows up certain excesses or deficiencies. Unfortunately each one also has its limitations. In this chapter we'll look at each test and help you decide which is best for you.

## Blood Testing

Blood is the most frequently used source of mineral information because it is quickly and easily extracted. Most doctors, when searching for causes of an illness which are not immediately apparent, will take a blood sample and send it to a laboratory for analysis. This sort of analysis can provide a complete biochemical profile of the blood. If requested by the doctor the blood levels of most of the body's vital minerals will be included in the results. However, these results are usually far from complete and in many cases can be downright misleading. Let's see why.

Firstly, while most minerals circulate in the blood and therefore leave discernible traces, they only use the blood as a quick and efficient way of getting to other parts of the body where they perform their main biochemical roles – the exceptions being iron and copper. This means that the amounts of minerals in the blood are often radically different from the amount found in those areas where they perform their primary functions. Judging cellular mineral levels by the amounts of minerals found in the blood is rather like estimating the population of a city by the number of cars on its roads. It is impossible and almost futile to judge it in this way.

Let's look at the example of calcium. Most of this mineral is contained in the bone and nerve cells rather than the blood and a series of regulatory hormones are used to keep its blood levels fixed within narrow limits. Therefore, from one cause or another, your bones and nerve cells may be catastrophically calcium deficient yet this deficiency won't show up in the blood test. Alternatively you might absorb a perfect amount of calcium while your magnesium levels are depressed. Since adequate magnesium is needed to stimulate the secretion of calcitonin – the bone-storing hormone – and suppress PTH – the bone-withdrawal hormone – this magnesium shortage will leave the calcium to circulate in the blood. The blood test will then reveal this elevated blood calcium and to pre-empt the danger of atherosclerosis and calcification of the soft tissue your doctor might recommend reducing your calcium intake, even though the calcium level was perfect. Remember, it was magnesium that was lacking not calcium which was excessive. Magnesium, however, is concentrated in the cells and, like calcium, a shortage is hard to discern by blood analysis.

Potassium is another problem nutrient when it comes to blood testing. It, too, is concentrated in the cells, leaving only trace amounts in the blood. High cellular potassium is often compensated for by low blood potassium. Yet, since a blood test is often the only diagnostic tool available, doctors often have to rely on the blood for a picture of the body's potassium levels. And because of this it may be a highly inaccurate picture.

Heavy metal toxicity also escapes diagnosis in blood testing. When the body ingests heavy metals such as lead and mercury, they are absorbed through the gut wall and circulated into the blood. However, their destructive oxidizing abilities quickly damage the numerous enzyme systems in the blood – enzymes that are used to transfer oxygen from the lungs to the cells, carry hormones, distribute nutrients and provide transport for the cells of the immune system. Naturally, the body will want to move these metals away from the blood as quickly as possible. It does this by stashing them in the bones, hair and nails. When a blood test is performed, therefore, it may show only negligible amounts of the heavy metals, suggesting to the doctor that the patient's body is relatively free of the toxins. In fact he might be suffering from a health-threatening excess.

Of course, for other minerals – those whose functions are performed primarily in the blood – this test is perfectly adequate. In particular, the levels of both iron and copper seem to be accurately reflected by blood tests.

## Urine testing

The analysis of urine samples is another commonly applied test for determining mineral levels. Like blood testing it can be misleading and inaccurate. For example, higher than normal levels of a particular mineral in the urine obviously show that the body is excreting this mineral in greater than normal quantities. The next question is why. The obvious answer is that it is excreting more than normal in order to reduce the body's levels of that mineral, possibly because it had ingested more than it needed. Yet this could be completely the wrong conclusion to draw. We've already seen with the calcium-magnesium relationship that an excess in the blood and urine may actually be caused by the fact that the mechanism which the body uses to store a particular mineral –thereby preventing this excess – is impaired. So here we have a situation where, thanks to the urine test, a mineral excess is diagnosed, when in fact the true problem might be that the cells are being depleted of the mineral.

Another failing common to both blood and urine analysis is that these tests can only represent the current condition of the body. Therefore, although the patient might be seriously deficient in a number of minerals, he will only be required to eat well over the few days prior to his tests to present a short-term picture of healthy mineral levels. The test that will provide a more accurate, comprehensive and longer-term mineral history is hair analysis.

## Hair Analysis

In his book, *Trace Elements, Hair Analysis and Nutrition*, Richard Passwater says that unlike blood, hair is 'permanently recording the past events of your trace elemental status'. Hair grows at the rate of about six inches a year. In doing so it gathers small amounts of almost every substance in the body – proteins, fatty acids, vitamins, minerals and heavy metals – and concentrates them into the shaft of the hair. The amount of a particular substance which is built into the hair depends on its availability. The smaller the amount contained in the body, the lower its levels in the hair. A single strand of hair, therefore, is like a constantly unfolding, continually updated story of your metabolism, providing a detailed picture of your body's health over many months.

Most of the research that has been conducted in this area concludes that hair is a much more accurate reflection of a large number of the body's mineral levels than either blood or urine. As the patient is required to do no more than contribute a snippet of hair, usually from the lower part of the neck, it is a simple, non-invasive test. It is particularly accurate at detecting heavy metal toxicity. Hair mercury levels, for example, are generally accepted as the best indicators for past exposure to mercury.

Of course, even though hair analysis presents a more comprehensive, longer-term mineral profile, certain factors do need to be taken into account when it comes to interpreting the results. It really comes down to sensitivity towards the numerous interrelated functions of the body together with a little elementary detective work. If all the minerals in the hair are low then you can infer that either you are not eating enough good mineral foods, or that you suffer from poor digestion. On the other hand, elevated levels of a single mineral such as calcium may indicate calcium loss from the bone and cells. Health practitioners will then have to look for metabolic causes of this rise in calcium rather than simply restricting intake. It may, for example, help to confirm the symptoms of low magnesium intake. In the same way, raised zinc levels may be due to so little zinc being available that hair growth slows down, thus making the zinc more concentrated.

You should also take into account any recent activities that are likely to have altered the composition of your hair. If you have been swimming in a pool your hair might contain elevated levels of copper thanks to the copper which had been added to the water to control algae. And higher than average levels of selenium might have resulted from using a shampoo such as Selsun. Bleaching your hair, on the other hand, is likely to denude it of certain minerals, particularly copper, zinc and manganese.

Finally, iron in the hair is an unreliable indicator of body stores and in this case at least a blood test is preferable. As you can see, hair analysis is only one part of a jigsaw puzzle that the trained practitioner must assemble in order to account for the problems of deficiencies and excesses.

## Saliva Analysis

Saliva analysis is a new form of testing under investigation by a small group of avant-garde nutritionists and researchers. Undoubtedly it will find its place in the world of mineral testing, suffering, like the others, from certain limitations, as well as possessing obvious advantages. For one thing it is less invasive and more convenient than either blood or urine testing. Like these two, though, saliva testing can only adequately reflect the current metabolic status of the patient, rather than give the more complete picture that hair analysis provides.

## Zinc

There is also a test designed specifically to determine the presence of zinc in the body. Professor Bryce-Smith has researched, developed and tested a liquid form of zinc that can be used as a taste-test. The patient is required to keep a small amount of this liquid in his mouth for about ten seconds and then to swallow it. Depending on how much zinc there is in the patient's body, his reaction will range from an inability to taste the liquid at all (signifying very low body zinc) to finding the liquid absolutely disgusting (meaning that the body levels of zinc are healthy). This test – known appropriately, as Zincatest – is only available from Nature's Best (see page 174 for address).

## Iodine

Another simple test for assessing the level of an individual mineral is the one devised by Dr Wright for determining adequate iodine levels. Using a bottle of tincture of iodine, obtainable from most chemists, simply paint a 5 cm square on the inside of your thigh before going to bed. Examine the area in the morning. If the square is still there your iodine stores are sufficient, but if it has disappeared then your body needs more iodine.

## Intracellular Testing

Unlike the other tests that we've looked at, an intracellular examination is not widely available and can be prohibitively expensive. This is a shame because it provides the patient with one of the most comprehensive mineral profiles possible. Basically, the test involves scraping a wooden spatula along the floor of the mouth under the tongue to remove some cells. These are placed on a glass slide and treated with a fixative solution to preserve their chemical identity. The slide is then put under an electron microscope which focuses on the composition of the cell, revealing the levels of many of the most important minerals. As far as we know, there is no laboratory in Britain which performs the test. If you'd like to find out more about it you should write to the American laboratory that has made this field its speciality. Its address is: Spectro-Scan, San Bruno Avenue, Suite 10, San Bruno, California 94066.

## CHAPTER 20

# Choosing Your Supplements

Having read in this book about the various causes and symptoms of mineral deficiency, you might realize that your body is lacking one or more of the mineral family. You may, for instance, have a recurring illness or disorder that has remained undiagnosed for years but which you now understand to be caused by a depletion. Alternatively, you may have discovered, thanks to a mineral profile of your hair, blood or urine, that you are the victim of certain dietary imbalances. Then again, you might simply want to increase your intake of particular minerals as a means of insuring yourself against the possibility of osteoporosis or circulatory problems occurring sometime in the future. If you want to improve your mineral intake for these or any other reasons, how should you go about it? The obvious answer is to reconstruct your dietary patterns on a balanced foundation of nutrients, including in what you eat a selection of foods that are rich in each and every essential mineral.

However, throughout this book we've seen cases which suggest that even were you to improve radically your diet you might still be at risk from a great many dietary variables. These render it almost impossible for you to assess accurately how much of each mineral you have been receiving. Pesticides, pollution, stress, viral infections and digestive difficulties, to name but a few, can all prevent you from ingesting all the vital minerals that you need from your diet. Therefore, you may decide to start taking mineral supplements. Unfortunately, even this isn't as simple as it sounds. Most good nutritional supplement manufacturers and health shops stock a variety of different mineral forms, and while the choice is by no means as wide as it is of vitamin supplements you are still faced with a bewildering variety when you try to decide which are right for you. This chapter aims to clarify things.

The most important question to ask when you choose mineral supplements is not how many of a particular tablet or pill you should take, or how many tablets or pills are contained in each canister, but rather how bio-available they are. Bio-availability is a measure of the degree of ease with which the mineral is absorbed across the gut wall as well as its solubility in the body. Most minerals are sold in several different forms and their bio-availability varies widely. Obviously you want to choose the most thoroughly absorbed mineral you can, so which one should you go for?

## The Claw Element

At the start of the book we drew the distinction between organic and inorganic substances. Organic substances, you may remember, are the living, regenerating substances such as proteins, vitamins and fatty acids, whereas inorganic substances are the eternally unchanging minerals. However, when it comes to the way that these substances are used as part of the body's biochemical mechanism their divisions start to blur. For even though the minerals themselves are inorganic, the body is best able to absorb them when they are bound up with a protein or a salt into an organic form. In Chapter 4 we mentioned the importance of vitamin D for absorbing calcium. Vitamin D is needed because it stimulates the production of a protein which latches onto the calcium and carries it across the gut wall into the body. The more vitamin D we eat, or manufacture from sunlight, the more calcium we can absorb from our food (of course, this doesn't necessarily mean that the calcium will be utilized properly once in the body).

The process whereby protein is used to bind to a mineral and carry it into the body in a metabolic piggy-back, is called chelation, which means 'to form a claw'. Chelation, in fact, works in either direction. There is a medical process called chelation therapy which involves injecting a patient with a highly active amino acid called EDTA. This amino then scours the body, latches onto toxic heavy metals such as lead and mercury, removes them from the cells and excretes them in the urine. Sadly, EDTA also has a tendency to remove essential nutrients such as zinc and should only be used under the strictest supervision.

However, for our purposes chelation is an excellent way of ensuring that the body absorbs its minerals as effectively as possible. Chelated minerals, in fact, are usually described as 'organic' because of their protein bond, or because they have formed a salt compound. Often you'll see a mineral supplement canister with the words 'amino acid chelated' on the label, which means that a number of amino acids have been used in the process. On other occasions manufacturers will use a single amino acid such as aspartic acid or methionine, both of which are excellent chelators. Other forms of minerals generally available include the gluconates, a good organic salt form, and the ascorbates, which are the mineral forms of ascorbic acid, otherwise known as vitamin C. Both these forms are well absorbed by the body. On the other hand, the widely available mineral salts such as the carbonates and phosphates are generally not so well absorbed. Finally, at the bottom of the mineral supplement tree come those minerals which, although organic, are obtained from the structural components of organisms. These include bone meal and oyster shell and are very much more difficult to absorb.

## Mineral Supplement Guide

This guide is by no means comprehensive but includes those supplements which we think provide the best value in terms of bio-availability.

### *Calcium*

| | |
|---|---|
| Calcium ascorbate | A calcium form of vitamin C. Very well absorbed and transported into the body. |
| Calcium aspartate | An amino acid chelate that is well absorbed and transported. |
| Calcium orotate | An acid form that enhances absorption in the gut. |
| Calcium gluconate | A salt derived from glucose. Absorbed and transported well. |
| Calcium lactate | A salt derived from lactic acid. Absorbed and transported well, although not advisable if you suffer from lactic intolerance. |
| Bone meal | Bone obtained from animals working in, or slaughtered near, an industrial environment may contain dangerous levels of lead. Ensure your bone meal comes from South America rather than North America or Europe. It has low calcium potency and is absorbed with difficulty, particularly by those suffering from low stomach acid. |
| Calcium carbonate | Poorly absorbed, particularly by the elderly or those suffering from low stomach acid. |

### *Chromium*

As chromium's sole function in the body is to assist insulin in storing and releasing glucose for energy production, the best way to obtain it is in its active form as Glucose Tolerance Factor (GTF). It is also available as an amino acid chelate.

### *Copper*

The body is usually able to absorb copper easily and any form is liable to be effective. Good forms include copper sulphate, copper gluconate and copper as an amino acid chelate.

### *Iodine*

| | |
|---|---|
| Seaweed or kelp | A natural, easily absorbed and rich source. |
| Potassium iodide | Laboratory-created but easily absorbed nonetheless. |

### *Iron*

Iron should be obtained from food sources rather than from supplementation. Only in rare, acute cases is there really a need for iron supplementation. Most forms are well absorbed. (A list of iron-rich foods is on p. 88.)

| | |
|---|---|
| Ferrous gluconate | Iron combined with glucose-derived gluconic acid. |
| Ferrous carbonate | An inorganic form. |
| Ferrous sulphate | An inorganic form. |
| Amino acid chelate | An iron molecule bonded with an amino acid to ensure the best possible absorption through stomach lining. |

### *Magnesium*

| | |
|---|---|
| Magnesium ascorbate | A magnesium form of vitamin C. Very well absorbed and transported. |
| Magnesium aspartate | An amino acid chelate that is absorbed and transported well. |
| Magnesium orotate | An acid form that enhances absorption in the gut. |
| Magnesium gluconate | A glucose-derived salt. Absorbed and transported well. |
| Magnesium sulphate | Good, but may cause diarrhoea. |

### *Manganese*

No form of manganese is easily absorbed, but the best available are:

| | |
|---|---|
| Manganese gluconate | A glucose-derived salt. |
| Manganese glycinate | An amino acid chelate. |

*Potassium*

| | |
|---|---|
| Potassium gluconate | A gluconic acid-derived salt. Easily absorbed. |
| Potassium aspartate | An amino acid chelate. |

*Selenium*

| | |
|---|---|
| Selenate and/or Seleno-methionine | These two forms of selenium – salt and chelate – should be taken together for maximum effect. |

*Zinc*

| | |
|---|---|
| Zinc citrate | A form of citric acid. Very well absorbed. |
| Zinc piccolinate | A form of piccolinic acid. Very well absorbed. |

(See also Zincatest in Chapter 19.)

**Suppliers**

Most good health food shops should stock a selection of minerals. Be wary of the bottles or canisters that fail to detail the form of the mineral which they contain. If you're unable to find a mineral supplement that you feel confident of using, the suppliers listed below should be able to meet your needs.

Cantassium
Larkhall Laboratories
225 Putney Bridge Road
London SW15
(01) 870 0971

G. R. Lane
Sissons Road
Gloucester

Natural Flow
Burwash Common
East Sussex
(0435) 882482

Nature's Best
P.O. Box 1
Tunbridge Wells
Kent TN2 3EQ
(0892) 34143

Nature's Own
Cheltenham
Glocs. GI50 1HX

Quest Vitamins
Unit 1
Premier Trading Estate
Dartmouth Middleway
Birmingham B7 4AT

# References

asterisk indicates that the reference is used in more than one chapter

**Chapter 1**

Anabolic Foods Inc. *Techni-Briefs*, Irving, California

*The Biochemical Role of Chelated Minerals in Maintaining Optimal Body Biological Functions*, International College of Applied Nutrition, June 1976

Chatsworth C. and L., 'Energy', *Healthview*, Charlottesville, Virginia, 1985

Hoffer A., *Orthomolecular Nutrition*, Keats, Connecticut, 1978

'Intoxication', *Annals of Rheumatic Disease*, no. 44, 1985

Kutsky R., *Handbook of Vitamins, Minerals, and Hormones*, 2nd edition, Van Nostrand Reinhold Co, New York, 1981*

Lappe F., *Diet for a Small Planet*, Ballantine, New York, 1975

Mervyn L., *Minerals and Your Health*, Keats, Connecticut, 1978

Pfeiffer C., *Zinc and Other Micro-Nutrients*, Keats, Connecticut, 1978

Rose S., *The Chemistry of Life*, Pelican, London, 1985

Schroeder H., 'Trace Elements in Clinical Chemistry', *Clinical Chemistry*, Vol. 17, no. 6, 1971

Schroeder H., *The Trace Elements and Man*, Devin Adair, Connecticut, 1975

Weiser M., *Calcium: Absorption and Malabsorption of Mineral Nutrients*, Alan R, Liss, New York, 1984, 15–68

**Chapter 2**

Hildenbrad G., *The American Revolution in Cellular Biology Healing*, Vol. 2, no. 1, 1982

*Journal of the American College of Nutrition*, no. 4, 1985, 107–120

Mervyn L., *Minerals and Your Health*, Keats, Connecticut 1981*

Basswater R., *Trace Elements. Hair Analysis and Health*, Keats, Connecticut, 1963

Schroeder H., *The Trace Elements and man*, Devin Adair, Connecticut, 1975*

**Chapter 3**

Adams R., *Minerals Kill or Cure*, Larchmont, N.Y.

Hildenbrad G., 'The American Revolution in Cellular Biology', *Healing*, Vol. 2, no. 1, 1982

*Journal of the American College of Nutrition*, no. 4, 1985, 107–120

Mervyn L., *Minerals and Your Health*, Keats, Connecticut, 1981*

Passwater R., *Trace Elements, Hair Analysis and Health*, Keats, Connecticut, 1963*

Schroeder H., *The Trace Elements and man*, Devin Adair, Connecticut, 1975*

**Chapter 4**
Adams R., 'Calcium Today?', *Better Nutrition*, Vol. 44, no. 6, June 1984
Albanese A. A., 'Calcium Nutrition in the Elderly', *Nutrition and the M.D.*, Vol. 5, no. 12, December 1979, 1–2
Avioli L., 'Calcium and Osteoporosis', *Annual Review of Nutrition*, 1984
Bickle D., 'Calcium Absorption and Vitamin D Metabolism', *Clinical Gastroenterology*, Vol. 12, no. 2, 1983
'Calcinosis of Joints and Periarticular Tissues Associated with Vitamin D Intoxication', *Annals of Rheumatic Disease*, no. 44, 1985
'Calcium, Bones and Teeth', *Prescribing Biochemists Ltd.,* Dec. 1985
Cheung A., 'Calcium to Magnesium Ratio', *Quest Vitamins*, 1987
*Calcium*, Dartell Laboratories
*Felmore Newsletter*, 76, Tunbridge Wells
*Felmore Newsletter*, 93, Tunbridge Wells
Ford N, *Calcium the Youth Vitamin*, Bestways, Aug 1986
Gordon G., 'New Dimensions in Calcium Metabolism', *Osteopathic Annals*, Spring 1983
Grant E., *The Bitter Pill*, Corgi, London, 1986
Henry R., 'Calcium Nutrition and Bone Health in the Elderly', *American Journal of Applied Nutrition*
Kussar, R., ed. *Vitamin D*, Martinus Nijhoff Publishing, Boston
Hildenbrad G., 'The American Revolution in Cellular Biology', *Healing*, Vol. 1, no. 1, 1982*
McCarron D., 'Serum Ionized Calcium and Dietary Calcium', *Human and Experimental Hypertension; Phosphate and Mineral Metabolism*, Plenum Publishing, 1984
*Merck Manual*, 14th ed. Merck and Co., New Jersey, 1982
Miller J., 'Calcium's Protein Partner', *Science News*, Vol. 118, *Nutrition and Health*, Vol. 6, no. 1, 1984, Columbia University, Aug 1980
Nordin B. E. C., *Calcium, Phosphate, and Magnesium Metabolism*, Churchill Livingstone, Edinburgh, London and N.Y., 1976
Rose S., *The Chemistry of Life*, Pelican, London 1985*
Spencer, H., 'Calcium Requirements in Humans', *Basic Science and Pathology*, no. 184, April 1984
Spencer H., *Effect of Certain Minerals on the Bioavailability of Calcium in Adult Males*, Veteran's Administration Hospital, Illinois, 1985
Weiser M., *Calcium; Absorption and Malabsorption of Mineral Nutrients*, 15–68, Alan R. Liss, New York, 1984

**Chapter 5**
Adams R., 'Calcium Today?' *Better Nutrition*, Vol. 44, no. 6, June 1984*
Bengoa J., *Magnesium*, 69–88
Cheung A., 'Calcium to Magnesium Ratio', *Quest Vitamins*, 1987*
*Felmore Newsletter*, 76, Tunbridge Wells*
*Felmore Newsletter*, 93, Tunbridge Wells*
*The Merck Manual* 14th Edition, Merck and Co., New Jersey, 1982*

Nordin B. E. C., *Calcium, Phosphate, and Magnesium Metabolism*, Churchill Livingstone, Edinburgh, London and N.Y., 1976
Passwater R., 'Trace Elements', *Hair Analysis and Health*, Keats, Connecticut, 1983*
Pfeiffer C., *Mental and Elemental Nutrients*, Keats, Connecticut, 1975
Randell R. E. et. al., 'Magnesium Depletion in Man,' *Ann. Internal Med.* 50 (2) 257–287, 1959
Schroeder H. A., 'Essential Metals in Magnesium', *J. Chron. Dis.* 21 (11–12): 815–841, 1969
Seelig M. S., 'The Requirement of Magnesium by the Normal Adult', *Amer. J. Clin. Nutr.* 14 (6) 342–390, 1964
Seelig M. S., *Magnesium Deficiency in the Pathogenesis of Disease*, Plenum Publishing Co., New York, 1980
Trimmer E., *The Magic of Magnesium*, Thorsons, Wellingborough, 1987

**Chapter 6**

*Calcium, Bones and Teeth*, Prescribing Biochemists Ltd., December 1985*
Feldheim W., 'Relationship Between Calcium and Phosphorus in Human Nutrition', *Milchwissenschaft*, Vol. 38, no. 5, 1983
*Felmore Newsletter*, 93, Tunbridge Wells*
Gordon G., 'New dimensions in Calcium Metabolism,' *Osteopathic Annals*, Spring 1983
Hildenbrand F., 'The American Revolution in Cellular Biology', *Healing*, Vol. 2, no. 1, 1982*
Nordin B. E. C., *Calcium, Phosphate, and Magnesium Metabolism*, Churchill Livingstone, Edinburgh, London and N.Y. 1976
Spencer H., *Effect of Certain Minerals on the Bioavailability of Calcium in Adult Males*, Veteran's Administration Hospital, Illinois, 1985*

**Chapter 7**

Boyd E. M., 'The Acute Oral Toxicity of Sodium Chloride', *Arch. Intern. Pharm. et Ther.* 144, 86–96, 1963
Dahl L. K., 'Role of Dietary Sodium in Essential Hypertension', *Jour. Amer. Dietic Ass.* 34, 585–590, 1958
Dahl L. K., 'Influence of Dietary Potassium and Sodium Molar Ratios on the Development of Salt Hypertension', *J. Exp. Med.*, 136, 318–330, 1972
*Felmore Newsletter*, 93, Tunbridge Wells*
Kutsky R., *Handbook on Vitamins, Minerals and Hormones*, 2nd edition, Van Nostrand Reinhold, N.Y., 1981
Leiter L., 'Low Sodium Syndrome: its Origins and Varieties', *Bull. N.Y. Acad. Med.* 29 (11) 833–845, 1953
*Nutrition and Health*, Vol. 6, no. 1, Columbia University, 1984
*Nutrition Almanac*, McGraw Hill, New York, 1979
Pearson D., *Life Extension*, Warner Books, New York
Polunin M., *Minerals*, Thorsons, Wellingborough, 1986

**Chapter 8**

Bryce-Smith C., *The Zinc Solution*, Century, London, 1987
Buchanan W.M., 'Iron Overload', *Cent. Afr. J. Md.* 18 (92) 35–40, 1972

Dowdy R.P., 'Copper Metabolism,' *Amer. J. Clin. Nutr.* 22 (7) 887–892, 1969
Dugdale A. E., 'Acute Iron Poisoning, Its Effects and Treatment', *Med. J. Australia* 51 (25) 990–992, 1964
*Felmore Newsletter*, 77, Tunbridge Wells
Hallberg L., 'Iron Absorption and Iron Deficiency: Human Nutrition', *Clinical Nutrition* no. 36, 259–278, 1982
Kell H.L., 'Role of Copper in Haemoglobin Formation,' *Jour. Biol. Chem.* 93 (1) 49–57, 1931
Kuhn I., 'Iron Absorption in Man', J. Lab. Clin. Med. 71 (5) 715–721, 1968
Kutsky R., *Handbook of Vitamins, Minerals and Hormones*, 2nd edition, Van Nostrand Reinhold, N.Y. 1981
Passwater D., *Trace Elements, Hair Analysis and Health,* Keats, Connecticut, 1983*
Pfeiffer C., *Zinc and other Micronutrients*, Keats, 1978
Pfeiffer C., *Mental and Elemental Nutrients*, Keats, Connecticut, 1975*
Polunin M., *Minerals*, Thorsons, Wellingborough, 1986*
Sternlieb I., 'Absorption of Copper in Malabsorption Syndromes' *J. Clin. Invest.* 43 (6) 1049–1055, 1964
Turnberg L. A., 'Excessive Oral Iron Therapy Causing Haemochromatosis', *Brit. Med. J.* 5446, 1360, 1965
Wintrobe M. M., 'Studies on Function and Metabolism of Copper,' Jour. Nutr. 50 (4) 395–420, 1953

**Chapter 9**
Adams R., *Minerals: Kill or Cure*, Larchmont, New York, 1975*
Kutsky R., *Handbook of Vitamins, Minerals, and Hormones*, 2nd edition, Van Nostrand Reinhold, N.Y., 1982
Mervyn L., *Minerals and Your Health*, Keats, Connecticut, 1981
North B. B., 'Manganese Metabolism in college women', *Jour. Nutr.* 72 217–223, 1960
Polumin M., *Minerals,* Thorsons, Wellingborough, 1987*
Rubenstein A. H., 'Manganese-Induced Hypoglycemia' *Lancet* 1348–1351, 1962
Schroeder H., 'Trace Elements in Clinical Chemistry', *Clinical Chemistry* Vol. 17, no. 6, 1971*

**Chapter 10**
Adams R., *Minerals: Kill or Cure*, Larchmont, New York, 1975*
Hoffer A., *Orthomolecular Nutrition*, Keats, Connecticut, 1985
Kenton L., *Ageless Ageing*, Century, London, 1986
Kutsky R., *Handbook of Vitamins, Minerals, and Hormones*, 2nd edition, Van Nostrand Reinhold, N.Y., 1982
Passwater R., *Selenium as Food and Medicine*, Keats, New York
Pearson D., *Life Extension*, Warner Books, New York, 1982*
Wallach S., 'Clinical and Biochemical Aspects of Chromium Deficiency', *Journal of the American College of Nutrition*, no. 4, 1985

**Chapter 11**
Diamond E., 'Vanadium Excretion, Toxicity, Lipid Effect on Man' *Am. J. Clin. Nutr.*, 12, 49–53, 1963

Hopkins L., 'Vanadium as an Essential Nutrient', *Fed. Proc. Fed. Am. Soc. Exp. Biol.*, 1974
Hudson T., *Vanadium Toxicology and Biological Significance*, Elsevier, London, 1964, 55–71
Kutsky R., *Handbook of Vitamins, Minerals and Hormones*, 2nd ed., Van Nostrand Reinhold Co., 1981
*Trace Elements in Human and Animal Nutrition*, 4th Ed., Academic Press, N.Y. 1976

**Chapter 12**

Asai K., *Germanium*, 1984
'Germanium', *Here's Health*, April 1987

**Chapter 13**

Cheraskin E., 'Prevalence of Possible Lead Toxicity as determined by Hair Analysis', *J. Orthomol Psych.*, Vol. 8, no. 2, 1977
Gordon G., 'Lead: Clinical Considerations,' *Osteo. Med.*, Vol. 3, no. 5, May 1978
'Hazards in Dentistry: The Mercury Debate', Kings College Cambridge, July 1985 *British Dental Soc. for Clin. Nutr.*
Hunter D., 'Cadmium Poisoning' *Arh. Hlg. Rada* 5: 221, 1954
Kark P. et al, 'Mercury poison and its Treatment', *N. Engl. J. Med.* 285 (1), 10–16, 1971
*Lead Intoxication in Children*, University of San Diego, 1985
Nath R., 'Molecular Basis of Cadmium Toxicity; Progress in Food and Nutrition', *Science*, Vol. 8, 109–163, 1984
Nordberg G., 'Cadmium Metabolism and Toxicity', *Environ Physiol Biochem* 2: 7, 1972
Peereboom-Stegeman J. H. J. C., 'Exposure and Health Effects of Cadmium', *Toxicological and Environmental Chemistry Reviews* Vol. 4, 671–678, Gordon and Breach Science Publishers Inc., 1981
Passwater R., 'Trace Elements,' *Hair Analysis and Health,* Keats, Connecticut, 1983
Revis N. W., 'Atherosclerosis and Hypertension Induction by Lead and Cadmium Ions: an Effect Prevented by Calcium Ions', *Proceeding of Natl. Acad. Sc.*, Vol. 78, no. 10, 6494–6498
Russell-Manning B., *Candida: Silver Fillings and the Immune System*, Greensward Press, San Francisco, Ca, 1986

**Chapter 14**

Harvey S., 'Heavy Metals', Chap 46, *Pharmacological Basis of Therapies*, L. Goodman, 1970
Mayo G. H., 'Aluminium, Absorption and Distribution: Effect of Parathyroid Hormone', *Science*, Vol. 197, 1977, 1187–1189
Schroeder H. A., 'Health Food Supplements Prepared from Kelp; A Source of Elevated Urinary Arsenic', *J. Chronic Dis.* 19, 85, 1966

**Chapter 15**

Albanese A. A., 'Bone Loss: Causes, Detection, and Therapy', *Current*

*Topics in Nutrition and Disease*, Vol. 1, Alan R. Liss Inc., New York, 1977
*Calcium, Bones and Teeth*, Prescribing Chemists Ltd., December 1985
Bickle D., 'Calcium Absorption and Vitamin D Metabolism', *Clinical Gastroenterology*, Vol. 12, no. 2, 1983*
Cheung A., *Calcium to Magnesium Ratio*, Quest Vitamins, 1987
Cheung A., *Osteoporosis and Its Management*, Quest Vitamins, 1987
Felheim W., 'Relationship Between Calcium and Phosphorus in Human Nutrition', *Milchwissenschaft*, Vol. 38, no. 5, 1983*
*Felmore Newsletter*, 76, Tunbridge Wells*
Flink E., 'Magnesium Deficiency in Human Subjects – A Personal Historical Perspective', *Journal of the American College of Nutrition*, no. 4, 17–31, 1985*
Gordon G., 'New Dimensions in Calcium Metabolism', *Osteopathic Annals*, Spring 1983
Grant E., *The Bitter Pill*, Corgi, London, 1986*
Hausman P., *The Calcium Bible*, Sidgwick and Jackson, London, 1986
Korcak M., 'Add Exercise to Calcium in Osteoporosis Prevention', *Medical News*, JAMA Vol. 247, no. 8, 1982
Mayes K., *Brittle Bones and the Calcium Crisis*, Thorson, Wellingborough, 1987
'Perspective', *Journal of the American College of Nutrition*, no. 4, 17–31, 1985
Henry R., 'Calcium Nutrition and Bone Health in the Elderly', *American Journal of Clinical Nutrition**
Kussar R. ed., *Vitamin D,* Martinus Nijhoff Publishing, Boston
Talmage R.V. et al., 'Calcium Regulating Hormones', *Proceedings of the Fifth Parathyroid Conference, Oxford*, U.K., July 1974, Elsevier Publishing Co., N.Y.
Trimmer E., *The Magic of Magnesium*, Thorsons, Wellingborough, 1987*

**Chapter 16**

Daykin P., 'Stomach Acid and Megavitamins', *Orthomolecular Psychiatry*, Vol. 5, no. 3, 1976
Erdmann R. and Jones M., *The Amino Revolution,* Century, London, 1987*
Hunt J., 'Relation Between Gastric Secretions of Acid and Urinary Excretion of Calcium After Oral Supplements of Calcium', *Digestive Diseases and Science*, Vol. 28, no. 5, May 1985
*Lead Intoxication in Children*, University of San Diego, 1985*
Pfeiffer C., *Zinc and Other micro-Nutrients*, Keats, New York, 1978*
Weiser M., *Calcium: Absorption and Malabsorption of Mineral Nutrients*, 15–68, Alan R. Liss, New York, 1984*

**Chapter 17**

Adams R., *Minerals: Kill or Cure* Larchmont, New York, 1975
Flink E., 'Magnesium Deficiency in Human Subjects – A Personal Historical Perspective', *Journal of the American College of Nutrition*, no. 4, 17–31, 1985*
Golden M., 'Trace Elements in Human Nutrition', *Human Nutrition: Clinical Nutrition*, no. 36, 185–202, 1982*
Hallberg L., 'Iron Absorption and Iron Deficiency', *Human Nutrition: Clinical Nutrition*, no. 36, 259–278, 1982

McCarron D., 'Serum Ionized Calcium and Dietary Calcium in Human and Experimental Hypertension', *Phosphate and Mineral Metabolism*, Plenum Publishing, 1984*

Pfeiffer C., *Mental and Elemental Nutrients*, Keats, Connecticut, 1975*

**Chapter 18**

Erdmann R. and Jones M., *The Amino Revolution*, Century, London, 1987

Passwater R. and Trace Rose S., *The Chemistry of Life*, Pelican, London, 1985*

**Chapter 19**

Bryce-Smith C., *The Zinc Solution*, Century, London, 1987

Cranton E., 'Standardization and Interpretation of Human Hair for Elemental Concentrations', *J. Holistic Med.*, Vol. 4, no. 1, 1982

Mineralab Inc., *Nutrition by Computer Analysis*, Mineralab, 1978

Passwater R., *Trace Elements, Hair Analysis and Health*, Keats, Connecticut, 1983*

Yokel R. A., 'Hair as an Indicator of Excessive Aluminum Exposure', *Clin Chem*, Vol. 28, no. 4, 1982, 662–665

# Index

Page numbers in *italic* refer to the illustrations